LEAVING TINKERTOWN

Literature and
Medicine Series

STATEMENT OF PURPOSE: The art of writing and the science of
medicine offer very different approaches to some of the most intense
and mysterious human experiences. The Literature and Medicine
series, jointly sponsored by the University of New Mexico Press
and the University of New Mexico's Health Sciences Center, brings
together these two ways of understanding. Comprising fiction and
creative nonfiction, the series showcases stories that explore the nature
of health and healing and the texture of the experience of illness.

ADVISORY EDITORS: Elizabeth Hadas, Frank Huyler, MD, and
David P. Sklar, MD

LEAVING TINKERTOWN

Tanya Ward Goodman

University of New Mexico Press | Albuquerque

Portions of the book have been previously published:
The chapter "Moving Grandma West" appeared in a different version *A Cup of Comfort for Courage,* edited by Colleen Sell, Adams Media F+W Publications, 2004. The chapter "The Bird House" appeared in a different version *A Cup of Comfort for Families Touched by Alzheimer's,* edited by Colleen Sell, Adams Media F+W Publications, 2008.

Library of Congress Cataloging-in-Publication Data
Goodman, Tanya Ward, 1968–
  Leaving Tinkertown / Tanya Ward Goodman.
    pages cm
  ISBN 978-0-8263-5366-5 (pbk. : alk. paper) — ISBN 978-0-8263-5367-2 (electronic)
  1. Ward, Ross, 1941–2002. 2. Alzheimer's disease—Patients—Biography.
  3. Alzheimer's disease—Patients—Family relationships. 4. Fathers and daughters.
  5. Folk artists—United States—Biography. 6. Tinkertown Museum. 7. Goodman,
  Tanya Ward, 1968– —Family. I. Title.
  RC523.W357G66 2013
  616.8'310092—dc23
  [B]
            2013005317

For my family with boundless love and gratitude.

CONTENTS

Acknowledgments

DAVID, THEO, AND SADIE, you have my heart. Huge love for Mom, La, Eric, Jason, Megan, Hedy, Sandy, Jane, Olga, and Steven. I am proud to be part of your family.

Thanks to Sam Dunn, who convinced me to stop calling it a "project" and start calling it a "book"; and to Betsy Amster, the most untiring and supportive of agents. Thanks to the women of the "Olio" writers' group: Harron Kellner, Mona Gable, Joyce Fidler, and Bonnie Reich; and to the excellent writers Elizabeth Aquino, Denise Emanuel Clemen, Linda Hunt, and Shanna Mahin. Thanks to Elizabeth Saveri, Mary Ore, Susan Howard, Brad Griffith, Alexis Jacks, and Vicki Mendoza, cheerleaders all. I am grateful to Mayra Orellana, Jerri Fenton, and Alicia Rhodes for their friendship and the care they lavished on my children while I worked on the book. Love and long-time admiration to Brian Herrera for shepherding the manuscript to Beth Hadas at the University of New Mexico Press and to Beth for her eager reception. And to my dad, Ross Ward, who is with me always.

If you would like more information about Alzheimer's disease, please visit the Alzheimer's Association at alz.org

With It

I WAS CONCEIVED IN A PICKUP CAMPER on the New Mexico State Fair Grounds when my parents were on the road with the carnival. They were carting around a freak show called World of the Weird along with a miniature wood-carved western town my father had made, known then as Folk Arts Village. At the end of the Albuquerque run, my mom packed up her bags and left my father to manage the rest of his life alone. She returned to her family home in Rapid City, South Dakota, where I grew secretly for several months. After six years of unprotected sex my parents had assumed that they could not have children. They figured that when they parted on that dusty lot in New Mexico, they would stay apart. Five months later, in March of 1968, they reconciled around my mother's round belly and set up housekeeping in Albuquerque.

Although they stopped traveling with the carnival full time, Dad still packed up his brush box and hit the road a dozen times or more each year to work as a showpainter. Sometimes he painted brand new rides like the Sea Dragon and the Flying Bobs in a factory in Wichita, Kansas, but most of the time he headed out to one dusty lot after the next to slap color on rides that had been kicking around the road season after season. Carny folks call this being "with it," which means that even if you're not on the road, the road is always with you.

On the day that I was born, my father was supposed to be driving a convertible down Central Avenue in Albuquerque, in a parade commemorating the one-hundredth anniversary of the end of the Navajo Long Walk. Instead of chauffeuring a Native American princess in a Cadillac, he piled Mom into his old, blue Ford pickup and hightailed it to St. Joseph's Hospital in downtown Albuquerque, where he paced the halls for thirty-two hours until I was cut from my mother's womb and handed over to the nuns who fed me sugar water and told my parents that I was the most beautiful baby they had ever seen. My father paid the hospital with two crisp thousand-dollar bills that he'd kept tucked into his boots as securely as I'd been tucked into my mama's belly. That was no surprise. My father always paid in cash.

A month shy of my first birthday, Mom and Dad bought a house. Though they often called it a cabin, the cinder-block structure was without notable detail save its location at the bottom of a steep gravel driveway in the shadow of the Sandia Mountains. My brother, Jason was born a year later, and he and I grew up in this house. Subject to the creative whims of my dad, the house grew with us. At five and a half, when I began making my first offerings to the tooth fairy, Dad created a mosaic of bones near the front door. In elementary school, while I struggled with the multiplication tables, Dad commenced building a geodesic dome on the roof of our living room. As I navigated the treacherous social terrain of middle school, Dad shrugged off the rules, mixed a batch of cement and began to build walls made out of beer bottles.

My parents split, my dad remarried, I got braces and glasses and a bad perm. I wore tennis-shoe roller skates and rainbow suspenders. I stopped playing the clarinet and took up theater. I researched the pros and cons of the death penalty for my high-school debate team and went to prom with one boy while lusting for another. I held slumber parties and played truth or dare. I studied for the SAT and looked at college catalogs and when I finally left this house, I felt I was grown.

Sandia Park   *   *December 1996*

I AM SITTING AT THE KITCHEN TABLE at home in New Mexico. The sun has disappeared behind the inky shape of the mountain, and dusky blue tree shadows stretch over the new snow in the yard.

I wrap my fingers around a mug of tea and bring it to my mouth, letting the minty steam warm my nose. Every so often, I can hear a muffled swoosh-thump as clumps of snow slide off the tin roof and into the yard.

It is a couple of days after Christmas, and tomorrow morning, in the company of my Jack Russell terrier, Wallace, I will make the thirteen-hour drive back to my apartment in Los Angeles. My name has been on the lease for only a few months and the one bedroom hardly registers as home.

I moved into the apartment after breaking up with my boyfriend of three years. Because he was making the big paychecks, he kept the big house. Where once my morning view included the distant island of Catalina, now my breakfasts are eaten while watching the wide, white underpants of my downstairs neighbor flap on the line. Though I've managed to get a series of assistant jobs in television production and even have a couple of produced freelance scripts under my belt, at twenty-eight, my career as a television writer seems to be stalled.

Working under the assumption that one day I'll land one of those high paying television gigs, I've racked up more than $20,000 on about ten different credit cards. Every time the phone rings, I get a tight feeling in my chest.

"I'm sorry, I'm not allowed to talk on the phone," I say before hanging up on the confused caller.

I shift my debt from one piece of plastic to the next to stay afloat, keep my fingers crossed and wait for my big break.

"I sure do envy you, kiddo," Dad says, sitting next to me. He pats his knee and my dog, Wallace, jumps onto his lap. "Out there in Hollywood. You've got everything."

"Yeah?" I say.

"You've got Knott's Berry Farm, Disney, Watts Towers . . . the Hollywood sign. You've got the biggest sign in the West, that's something," Dad says. "I sure wish I was going back with you."

"Why don't you, honey?" My stepmother, La, stands behind Dad and rubs his shoulders. She is wearing her traditional winter ensemble: blue jeans and a well-loved cashmere sweater over a purple turtleneck. She rakes her fingers through her short blonde hair and says, "Road trip. It'd be good for you."

"Dare I? Dare I?" Dad bellows. "Dare I take my life into my own hands and jump into the fiery seat of the hottest car this side of the Indianapolis 500?"

"My Honda would get a kick out of being called a 'hot car,'" I say.

La crosses to the bookshelf and grabs the big Rand McNally road atlas that Dad always refers to as "the family bible." She puts the map down in front of us. I tie my long, brown hair in a knot to keep it out of my face and lean over the crumpled pages on the table where Dad's thick pointer finger charts our course from Albuquerque to Los Angeles. We decide to stay off the interstate as much as possible, following Route 66 through the desert, before driving down into the City of Angels.

"Hollywood," Dad sings. "Da da da da da Hollywood . . ." He dances his hands up Wallace's back, ending in a good ear rub. The dog closes his eyes in appreciation.

"I'll make you a plane reservation for the trip back," La says.

"Whoa, there. A plane?" Dad says. "I'll just come back with The Kid."

"She lives in Los Angeles, honey," La says.

"Of course she does," Dad says. "I don't like airplanes is all I meant."

"You want to take the train?" La asks.

"A train? Now that's the way to travel," Dad says. "Like the circus, like the Old West. Take a train through the desert. Sleep on the train, see the country."

"Perfect," La says, picking up the phone to book a ticket.

It is at times like this, when her efficiency is in full flow, that I think the shortening of her name from Carla to La makes perfect sense. It's the pet name first bestowed by her father and now reserved for family and the people who know her best. We know that sometimes she moves so fast that there's barely enough time to give her the full two syllables.

La was our next-door neighbor before she became my stepmother, catching my dad's eye long before he divorced my mother. I remember her in bright tank tops under clay-spattered overalls, her long blonde hair billowing from beneath a bandana. One year for Father's Day, she took black-and-white photos of my brother, Jason and me and then helped us create pottery picture frames in her studio. It is only now that I think to wonder at the effect this project must have had on my mother.

I was in my first year of college when La told me never to get involved with a married man. "I know this seems weird coming from me," she said, "But I mean it. It worked out for your dad and me, but it never works out. I was lucky and that kind of luck is rare."

La married Dad just about a year after he and Mom divorced. I think it was partially the infidelity that drove Mom away, but I also think she needed to complete the move she started when I was swimming unknown in her belly. She didn't want to be "with it," and she could tell that Dad was never going to be without it. He was a born showman.

Dad had always wanted to run his own roadside attraction, and with La's encouragement, he built a permanent home for the miniature western town he'd been carting around in a trailer since before I was born. Tinkertown Museum opened when I was a sophomore in high school. That first year, we had just under one thousand visitors. Every couple of days a car would drive down the driveway and across the black rubber air hose that rang a bell inside the house. One of us would come out and collect a dollar and open the gate so that tourists could walk around in our front yard.

"Sell 'em a look," Dad said, repeating the sage wisdom of his mentor Roy Healy, once the proprietor of The Antique Car Museum in Rapid City, South Dakota. "That's all you need to do." He'd wrap an arm around me and dig his tickling fingers into my side. "I'm gonna set you up with a ten-cent show. Maybe a two-headed squirrel or a hairless dog. Who needs college when you've got a two-headed squirrel? Right, kid?"

The museum grew and grew. Dad built with what he had, recycled signs, plywood, old barn siding and bottles and cement. He built a room off the front of the house made of green beer bottles alternating with emerald-colored gallon wine jugs, before adding a series of undulating glass bottle walls to enclose our backyard. He mixed bottles with rocks from the surrounding hills and studded the cement in between with bits of broken pottery and rhinestone jewelry and marbles and toys. Our friends and neighbors started saving their bottles, and every few days we'd find a few brown paper grocery sacks filled with new "bricks" at the front door.

All through my high-school years, Dad added more rooms to the museum to house his miniature circus and his collection of mining tools. He built wooden cases to hold a sword collection and more than two hundred wedding cake couples he'd picked up in antique shops all over the country. He parked a chuck wagon under our oak tree and traded a couple of signs for a two-seated buggy. He built more bottle walls and welded metal cutouts of angels to old steam engine wheels, forming towering webs against the turquoise New Mexico sky. With the museum walls layered, twisting, and circling around it, the house I grew up in began to grow darker and darker. By the time I passed up the ten-cent show in favor of Northwestern University, most of the rooms stood all day in the dim half-light of a late winter afternoon.

Things Start to Get Weird * *December 1996*

LA SWEEPS LAST NIGHT'S SNOW off my car with a broom while I scrape frost off the windows. My fingers are numb. It's hard to imagine that by tomorrow, I'll be back in Los Angeles where the lawns are green and I'll need no more than a sweater to stay warm. Dad shifts from one foot to the next.

"Honey, do you have to pee?" La asks.

"Will you leave me alone?" Dad says, but he goes inside anyway.

La's eyes follow him up the walk and into the house. "It's good for him to get out. Good for us to have a break."

"Is everything all right?" I ask.

"Of course," La says. "Everything is great. It's winter, that's all. You know your dad hates the snow."

Our trip starts out well. I punch a Dwight Yoakam tape into the cassette player and we sing along to "Guitars and Cadillacs" as I drive through Tijeras Canyon, into Albuquerque and out toward the West Mesa. Wallace sleeps on Dad's lap. Our goal is Kingman, where we'll find a motel and eat dinner before heading on into Los Angeles the next day. Dad keeps the road atlas nearby, pulling it out every so often to check our route. He draws a couple of burros near the ghost town of Oatman, Arizona, and a small desert landscape near Chloride where over two dozen years ago, his friend Roy Purcell painted a mural on some rocks at the end of a long, bumpy dirt road.

Suddenly, he becomes agitated. "You're going too damn fast. Jesus, Tanya, slow down."

The change in Dad's voice startles me. I'm only going a couple of miles over the limit, but I ease my foot off the gas and glance over at him. "You okay?"

"I'm okay, I'm okay. Would you women stop asking me if I'm okay, already? You can all go to hell, okay?"

I've known Dad to be frustrated or impatient, but he is almost never this way with me. I'm surprised by the roughness of his voice. I'm also confused. Who are these women? Why are they worried? I want to ask him who he's talking about, but I don't want him to get angrier, so I swallow my own voice and try to focus on the road ahead.

Our last road trip was more than ten years ago, when Dad drove me to college in Illinois. He figured he'd make it a work trip and drop me at school before continuing on to Arkansas to paint a couple of showfronts. We thought the drive would take us a just over two days, but we were having such a good time, we spent four days traveling through Kansas, Nebraska, and Iowa, going out of our way to visit Amish villages and eat hot fudge sundaes at small roadside diners. When we finally made it to Chicago we drove through the biggest city I'd ever seen, past the glorious houses along Lake Shore Drive and into the upscale suburb of Evanston. We drove past the huge brick building that was my dorm. We looked out the window of the truck and admired the fall leaves and the view of the lake and the beautiful stone campus chapel with the enormous stained-glass windows, but we did not stop until we were far, far away from the place where we would have to unload all my suitcases and boxes. Neither one of us spoke, but we shared a wordless agreement that we were not ready to part.

"We got the lay of the land, right?" Dad asked.

"We're cowards," I said.

Dad just kept driving until, in some far north suburb of Chicago, he pulled the van up to the curb in front of a small park. Maples dropped leaves red as match tips on the lawn. A couple of kids in puffy jackets pumped their legs on the swing set. A flock of small birds flew in a twittering cloud from tree to tree. Right up to that second, I think we had both been caught up in the momentum of the trip. We'd spent the last four days doing pretty much what we'd been doing my whole life: making jokes, singing along to the radio and stopping to look at whatever caught our eye, but now, we had arrived. Dad and I had been a team for so long that I hadn't really stopped to consider that at some point we would have to say good-bye.

"This is something, isn't it," Dad said, resting his big hand on the back of my neck. I nodded. His green eyes, the same color as mine, were teary.

He gave my shoulder a squeeze and wiped his eyes with the back of his hand. "Shit. Well, let's do it."

I had to remind myself to breathe as we drove back to Northwestern. We pulled into a space in front of my dorm and made ten trips up four flights of stairs with all of my things. After our last trip, Dad hugged me quickly and left me sitting on my narrow twin bed. For the longest time, I sat, surrounded by all my boxes. The voices of strangers rang out in the hall, cars passed on the street below my window. Finally, I plugged my pink cassette player into the nearest outlet and rummaged around to find a pile of tapes. Before I left home, I had recorded many of the albums in Dad's collection, bringing Bob Dylan, Leonard Cohen, and Emmylou Harris to college with me. When I pushed play, the hiss and crackle of the vinyl brought the sounds of home into this unfamiliar place.

Later, Dad would write to tell me that he ran down the stairs, jumped in the truck, and didn't stop driving until he hit Arkansas.

"I was pretty blown out—as you know," he wrote. "Big changes—and you were right—we are both cowards—however, I prefer to call it 'fear of unknown!'"

Evanston, Illinois, was as unknown as the moon. Coasting on a wave of Dad's faith in me, I'd applied to Northwestern without so much as a single visit to Chicago. Now that I was here, my clothes seemed wrong, my worn mix tapes out of touch compared to my roommate's stacks of CDs. I had never been to Europe, never eaten sushi, never joined the crowd at an R.E.M. concert. In fact, I wasn't all that sure I had ever heard of R.E.M. At the big mixers and dorm parties, I tried to overpower my anxiety with wine coolers and big, red Solo cups of beer. I read and re-read Dad's letter. "Fear of the unknown," was reassuring. It was a phrase filled with possibility. The unknown *could* become known. Even from a distance, Dad put a good spin on things. Even from a distance, I felt his love.

When I look back at Dad, his eyes are peaceful. He shifts Wallace carefully on his lap and looks at me expectantly.

"This is fun," he says. "It's good to see you."

His mood is so changed, I want to ask if everything is okay, but I'm worried that he'll be angry again. He seems different to me—nervous and childlike. I haven't lived in Albuquerque in ten years, and so I wonder if I've missed the gradual changes that come with age.

I try to recall the last letter I've gotten from Dad or the last phone call when he's been the only one on the line. I realize that for a long time, my birthday cards have been signed in La's loopy handwriting and that on the telephone, La has been doing most of the talking. I look across at Dad and he looks away from me and out the window to the far horizon.

We drive through the red rock of Gallup and out across the Painted Desert. We pass cement dinosaurs advertising petrified wood and the Geronimo Trading Post where kids get a free arrowhead. In Winslow, I start singing the Eagles song "Take it Easy" and Dad joins in, but only for a minute. He rubs Wallace's ears between his thumb and forefinger, mumbling softly into the dog's brown fur.

At Dad's urging, we get out of the car in Two Guns, Arizona, and walk down into the ditch to get a look at a sign reading "Live Mountain Lions" on the side of what looks like an abandoned petting zoo.

"This used to be a heck of a roadside attraction," Dad says. "Of course now the whole damn place is cursed."

"Cursed how?"

"It's some scary shit. The guy who owned this place told me that he'd found out it was an old Indian burial ground—some kind of death cave. Anyone who spent any time here was in for it, big time. He warned me to stay away. The curse is real, just look at this place. It could have been great and for no reason, it just failed."

I look around. There are a couple of sad, old buildings and a junky campground up on a dusty hill. The wind is blowing about two-hundred miles an hour and there isn't a tree as far as the eye can see.

"The owner got real sick. Life-threatening stuff. Finally shot himself right over there."

I follow Dad's finger to a stone shack with a collapsing roof.

"Went right down into the death cave to do it. You can't blame the son-of-a-bitch," Dad says. He turns and heads back to the car. Wallace prances along beside him.

My hair is whipping around my head and I can feel the sting as grains of sand hit my face. Although Dad is a known bullshitter and teller of tall tales, his story leaves me with an uneasy feeling in the pit of my stomach.

We hit Kingman in the late afternoon. When I ask Dad where we should stay, he gets mad and tells me it doesn't matter. So I drive into a cheap motel right next to a Denny's and book a room for the night. Inside it smells like smoke and cleaning fluid. A painting of an old mill hangs over one bed; over the other there is just a nailhead and a lighter square of wallpaper. Dad sinks into an easy chair near the desk. I open my suitcase and put my dopp kit down near the sink. Wallace bounces from one bed to the other and back just as my brother, Jason, and I did on all the family vacations of my childhood.

When I look up again, Dad is asleep in his chair. I wonder if I should call La. It seems that the further we get from Tinkertown, the shakier Dad gets. His head nods forward, crushing his beard against his chest. His faded blue denim shirt seems to hang on him. He's lost weight. The beer belly that has been a constant for most of my life seems to have diminished, and the skin sags around the muscles of his forearms. I take a deep breath and head for the sink to splash water on my face.

A while later, we're at the Denny's next door to the hotel. I look up from my shiny menu to see Dad's eyes following a waitress who holds a tray filled with wine glasses.

"A glass of wine would be nice, wouldn't it?" he says. "You'd have a glass, wouldn't you?"

"Well, I don't know," I say. I hate the way his eyes light up when he sees these junky little glasses filled with cheap wine.

When our server shows up, he orders a plate of French fries and a glass of red.

"French fries? Are you gonna eat anything else?"

"What is your problem?" he growls.

I am embarrassed and quickly order a tuna sandwich and a glass of water. It isn't that I don't want a drink. I do. It has been a long day and Dad is freaking me out, but I see the value in keeping a clear head. When Dad's wine arrives, he downs it in two quick swallows. As he orders his next glass, I tackle my sandwich, hoping to get through dinner before he can order a third.

There have been other nights like this in my life, other nights spent watching my dad drink that left me feeling sad to the core. "Loosen up," Dad would say when I'd ask him to stop drinking. "For God's sake, Tanya, loosen up."

On a normal day, we could communicate volumes with a simple raised eyebrow, but the alcohol made our connection fuzzy and tentative. His sudden change would often catch me by surprise because he didn't drink all the time. I must have been around nine or ten when I started watching for the signs, trying to prepare myself to lose him a little. I memorized the walk, the way his knees went liquid and loose, and watched for the glitter in his eyes, moist and vague above the flush of his cheeks. Usually, it was the desperation that tipped me off. He'd pull into a gas station with a full tank and come out holding a six-pack in a brown bag, shrugging his shoulders and saying, "Well, what do you know, they've got beer in there."

After dinner, Dad stumbles across the parking lot and collapses on his bed. He starts to snore almost immediately and doesn't wake up. Not when I pull his boots off and not when Wallace jumps up next to him and licks his face. Again, I want to call La, but I'm not sure what to say. I feel like I've failed already by letting him have a drink, let alone three.

The next morning, Dad wakes up with a headache. He spends a long time in the bathroom and doesn't want to stop for breakfast.

"My belly is funny," he says. "I don't know why."

It could be the handful of French fries floating around in cheap plonk, I think, but I keep these thoughts to myself. Today we're headed out to visit Roy Purcell's murals in Chloride.

Because of Dad's enthusiasm for roadside attractions, all of our family vacations included dozens of side trips. We visited Simon Rodia's Watts Towers in Los Angeles and Calvin Black's surreal doll theater, Possum Trot, way out in the Mojave Desert. We saw aging ballerina Marta Beckett dance at the Amargosa Opera House in Death Valley. In South Dakota, we paid annual visits to Dr. Niblack's Wood-Carving Museum and were on a first-name basis with the owners of the Clock Museum in Colorado Springs. Watts Towers still stands, but many of the places we visited have disappeared. I wonder if their disappearance has begun to weigh on Dad, making him question his own place on the map.

Despite a few missed turns we manage to make it to the murals. Painted on the red rocks nearly four decades ago, "The Journey" depicts an old mining town as well as various goddess figures and desert landscapes.

"Is this something or what?" Dad says, standing back and shielding his eyes from the sun. "Old Roy really did it right. He just got it, you know. I envy him."

"Why?" I ask.

Dad gestures broadly at the paintings. "Look at all he accomplished. Look what he did."

"Yeah, thirty years ago. Look at what you've done. Look what you're still doing."

"I don't know," Dad sighs. "What have I done, really?"

Dad walks Wallace up closer to the murals. I stand back and watch him stare intently at the artwork. It isn't like him to downplay his accomplishments. He's the guy who at the slightest provocation will have visitors climbing a ladder to the roof of our house to take in the aerial view of "what started out as a four-room cabin and is now a twenty-two-room compound." He's the guy who painted the sign at Tinkertown that reads, "I did all this while you were watching TV."

It is dark when we finally hit the Los Angeles County line, but the highway is illuminated by the strip malls and car lots and big-box stores that line Interstate 10. We are smack in the middle of rush hour with a line of red brake lights snaking out in front of us. The car smells like dog breath and potato chips and we are tired and hungry.

"What is all this?" Dad grumbles.

"It's Los Angeles," I reply. "Traffic."

"This isn't L.A." Dad continues to look out the window. "This is just trash. What was I thinking coming out here?"

I call David on my cell phone and ask him to meet us at a restaurant near my apartment. We've only been dating a couple of months, and in the same way that my apartment doesn't feel like home, David doesn't feel like a boyfriend. Sometimes I call him my "lovely parting gift," as if my previous relationship were some kind of game show where I had failed to win a washer. I also call him my "young buck" because at twenty-three, he's five years my junior.

David has a clean, square jaw and hazel eyes shaped like teardrops. We met when we were both working as writers' assistants. I liked the way his biceps bulged under his T-shirts. I liked his hands with their ragged, bitten fingernails, and I liked the way he seemed attentive to the needs of everyone, but was still able to carry on with his own life. The first time he spent the night at my house, we kissed and talked and laughed until the sun came up and he had to go home to get contact lens solution. I was so happy I got up and made a tarte tatin to bring in to work. The writers demolished the gooey apple pastry, and when they wondered why I felt compelled to bake at such an early hour, David gave me a secret smile that made me want to crawl across the conference table and bite his neck.

An hour later, we finally arrive at my apartment. Dad runs up the stairs and into the bathroom while I start to unload the car. On my second trip up the steps, I find Dad leaning against the kitchen counter guzzling wine straight out of a bottle.

"Jesus Christ, what are you doing?"

"Will you just simmer down?" Dad says. "It's been a long trip. I'm having a drink."

I grab the bottle and pour the little bit remaining into the sink.

I pull Dad out of my apartment and down the street to the Tam O'Shanter Restaurant.

As Dad and I stumble through the restaurant door, I'm feeling as though we've been tossed up by a storm. David is waiting on a bench by the hearth in the nook they call "the Snug." He's wearing the blue-plaid flannel shirt I gave him for Christmas, and his hazel eyes shine like a calm sea. He stands and gives me a shy kiss before reaching out to shake Dad's hand.

"I've heard so much about you, Mr. Ward," he says.

"Mr. Ward?" Dad jeers, "Get a load of this kid." His knees are loose and his face is red. "I'm gonna hit the john."

As soon as Dad lurches into the bathroom, I start to cry. "I don't know what's going on," I say. "He's not like this." I explain about the wine tonight and the wine last night and the desperation and the anger.

"It'll be good to get some food into him," David says. "And maybe some coffee."

I marvel at this guy. At twenty-three he is more level-headed than I am. I lean into him and take a deep breath.

The night goes from bad to worse. Dad eats only a few French fries and manages to foil my attempts to keep him from drinking by pounding back a beer at the bar on one of his trips to the bathroom. He gets so drunk that he pulls our waitress onto his lap.

"Well, isn't he something," she says, patting his hand before hauling herself up.

"I am something, sweetheart," Dad responds.

I leave the waitress a twenty-dollar tip.

Back at my apartment, David and I try to convince Dad to sleep in my bed. Instead, he grabs a blanket from the couch and hunkers down in the middle of the living-room floor.

"This'll do me just fine," he says. "I'll sleep down here with old Wallace."

With David's help, I manage to pull Dad's boots off and get him into a sleeping bag. He is asleep in minutes.

"You're sure you're going to be all right?" David asks.

"He's sleeping. I'm just going to hope he wakes up different."

"Call me if you need anything. I mean it. I'll be here as fast as I can."

A part of me wants to grab David and hold him tight; wants to keep him from leaving me alone with Dad. Another part of me is glad he can be free of this. I can see all the craziness in my life rising up around me like the bottle walls around Tinkertown. David should run now, I think.

David grew up in a white two-story house on a tree-lined street in Larchmont, New York. There was a basketball hoop in the driveway and bicycles in the garage. His dad was a news producer and his mom was a schoolteacher. David played football and was the prom king and dated a cheerleader. His family rented a summer house in the Hamptons, and on special occasions his dad wore a navy sports coats and his mom set her hair.

In the living room of the house where I grew up there was a four-foot ebony carving of a naked headhunter and a stuffed moose head wearing a pair of wire-rimmed glasses. There was a wood-burning stove where my father periodically heated up a branding iron and seared his initials into the walls and floors. My mother sewed all my clothes, embroidered flowers onto my skirts and blouses, and overdyed my jeans in a bathtub of pink RIT dye. Looking for something different, I'd run my fingers over the glossy pages of the Sears catalog, turning down the corners to mark butter-colored wingback chairs, crisp pastel blazers and plaid skirts to be worn with white knee socks and patent leather shoes. I would close the bathroom door on the sounds of my mother's Moody Blues albums and practice the upper-crust accent and knowing look of Hayley Mills.

Though I started school at an artsy co-op, by second grade, I was able to convince my parents to send me to San Antonito Elementary, where the bright yellow school buses were lined up in the parking lot neat as a box of pencils. I liked having a desk and a cubby for my coat. Sure, the place was what my folks called "straight," but the routine of homeroom Pledge of Allegiance, the damp, clean feel of freshly mimeographed worksheets, and the anticipation of seeing my teacher, Mrs. Netz, resplendent in her daily pantsuit made sense to me.

When I was about eight or nine, unwilling to leave my education entirely in the hands of the state, Dad started pulling me out of school and taking me with him to experience life "on the road." In a carnival winter quarters in Coolidge, Arizona, I earned a dime each for painting the hooves of twenty merry-go-round horses and met a man weighing over five hundred pounds who was known as "Tiny." Another time, in Arkansas, Dad parked next to a sideshow called "Willy the Whale." While Dad worked, I curled up in the back of our van and breathlessly read of Jo's professor in *Little Women*. Soon, Alcott's words shut out the roar of the generator used to keep the ancient whale carcass in deep freeze.

We slept in flannel sleeping bags in the back of the truck and once spent the night inside the entrance tunnel of a fun house. I grew used to washing up in the grimy bathrooms of factories and fairgrounds, using turpentine to rid my arms and legs of paint spots and slathering it off with Goop, the thick gel cleanser favored by mechanics and ride boys. I met men with so many prison tattoos their faces and arms seemed green. Once in Arkansas, I shook hands with a real circus fat lady named Alice from Dallas. Dad was usually paid in a wad of cash, which he called a "ham sandwich," and kept in a brown paper bag under the seat of the truck.

I grew up knowing that if I walked down a midway anywhere in the country I could avoid the pitch by telling the "jointy" that I was "with it." I knew that when the show picked up and moved from one city to the next it was called a "jump," cotton candy was "floss," a crummy location on the lot was the "donniker spot," and to a true carny a merry-go-round would always be a "Jenny."

I was with it, but I wasn't sure I was for it. With books like T. H. White's *The Once and Future King*, Lucy Maud Montgomery's *Anne of Green Gables*, and *The Chronicles of Narnia* for guidance, I walked around the lot imagining verdant meadows and enchanted forests in place of the crushed soda cans and straw wrappers. I walked slowly, taking measured steps. In my mind, I was wearing a ball gown or at the very least, a proper shirtwaist. With concentration I could transcend my cut-off jeans and faded T-shirt with the iron-on transfer of Mr. Bill. I read and read, and all the while I willed myself to achieve the cleverness of Nancy Drew, the passion of Guinevere, the brilliance of Marie Curie, and the creative inspiration and drive of Anne Shirley.

I resist the urge to escape into a book as Dad's visit to Los Angeles becomes more and more difficult. Dad can't or won't make a decision. He doesn't care what we eat or where we go. He seems more interested in talking to Wallace than in talking to me. We decide to drive out to Simi Valley to visit what is left of Grandma Prisbrey's bottle village, but he has such a hard time reading the map, I have to stop at three different gas stations to get directions. By the time we arrive he is so angry, he will barely speak to me. Once we get walk up to the chain-link fence surrounding the remains of Tressa Prisbrey's bottle houses, he seems to forget all about his anger.

"I'm sure glad you got to see this place when it was working," he says.

We met Grandma Prisbrey back in the '80s when she was already very,

very old. She gave us a personal tour of what she called her Bottle Village and told us how she'd found everything in the dump and turned it into something real nice. What I remember most about the tour was the huge black widow spider that scrambled out of the way as she reached to point out the largest pencil in her pencil collection, which was more than three feet long and as thick as my wrist.

Dad leans his face close to the fence and shouts a hello.

"Anybody there?" he shouts. "It's Ross Ward."

A woman appears. "Ross?" she says, coming forward. "Oh, Ross, bless you."

The woman, it turns out, is the caretaker. She and my dad have been exchanging letters for years.

"Your dad is a generous soul," she says. "It's on account of kind people like him that we haven't been bulldozed already." She invites us in and lets us wander around in the ruins. There are a few scaffolds set up around the broken buildings and a wheelbarrow encrusted with cement. After Grandma Prisbrey's death, many of the bottle buildings were damaged in the 1994 Northridge earthquake and the place was closed indefinitely for restoration.

"It looks like you're making some progress," Dad says gently. "It's really starting to come together."

The woman looks up at him, her eyes shining. "You think so?"

"I do," he says. He reaches into his back pocket and pulls out his wallet. He peels off a couple of twenties and presses them into her hand.

"Just keep building," he says. "It's going to be okay."

"You're kind of a celebrity," I say to Dad in the car on the way home. "That woman opened the gate as soon as she heard your name."

"She's a nice old gal," Dad says. "She's working really hard out there. It's just a shame she has to do it all by herself."

"It was nice of you to help her."

"That's all we can do," Dad says, reaching across and squeezing my knee. "Just help each other out now and then."

Within two blocks, Dad falls asleep and at every stoplight, I steal a glance. He's still out when I park in front of my apartment and so I really take him in. I see the familiar laugh wrinkles around his eyes and the way his hair falls across his forehead. He looks calm, and it is easy to think he might wake up right now and make a silly joke or tell me a story. It is easy to believe he might apologize for being so angry and strange. "Whew, that was something," he might say. "Crazy times, right?" But this isn't going to happen. Change is blowing in the air like so much desert sand. Something is wrong with Dad, but I don't know what. I blink my eyes hard against the tears.

That evening, at Union Station, we are both so tired we don't talk much. I want to apologize for being angry. I want to test him and ask him what he remembers from the last few days. I also want to get away. Dad seems to sense this.

"You don't need to hang around," he says. "I'm good."

"Are you sure?"

"I've got my ticket. The train is right there. I get on, right?" He smiles at me.

"Right. You can do it."

"I can do a lot," he says.

I hug him and he hugs me back, hard.

"Why are you crying?" he asks when I pull back.

"I hate good-byes," I say.

He gives me a wave and I walk away. At the door, I look back to see him sitting in one of the leather chairs. His shoulders are rounded, and he is staring straight ahead. I wave and push through the revolving door. The night air feels like a cool palm against my forehead.

Circling the Wagons ∗ *April 1997*

IT IS SPRING in New Mexico, which means the temperature can range twenty degrees on either side of sixty, often in the same hour. On bad days, the wind picks up and blows tumbleweeds, dust, and empty paper cups across the roads, filling the sky with a brown dirt haze. But on good days, when the sun is out and the sky is the clean blue of a robin's egg, I can think of no other place I'd rather be.

I am here to help La take Dad to the doctor. It took me three months and countless phone calls after I put Dad on the train in Los Angeles to screw up the courage to ask her whether she thought there might be something wrong with him.

"Oh, God, Tanya, I thought I was going crazy," La said. She told me that she'd been feeling it for months, but Dad got angry every time she brought it up. He'd been giving the wrong change in the museum gift shop and misplacing the keys to the car. He'd forgotten how to work the cash register and let his best sign-painting brushes harden in a can of paint.

My brother Jason, his fiancée Megan, La, and I hold a whispered pow-wow in the kitchen of the cottage while watching Dad through the window. He is gluing pennies to the hood of the old red Jeep Cherokee that he's started to call his "art car."

"I'm getting married," Jason tells us. "This is a big life change. I want to go into this knowing that everyone is okay."

Though he is two years younger, my tall, dark-haired brother has reached yet another milestone before me. He took his first drink before me, shared his first kiss before I did, lost his virginity years before I did, and now he's found his true love. I can see why he loves Megan. Smart and creative, she looks at the world through wide, blue eyes, above which carefully shaped brows gather to register curiosity, compassion, and pique. She guards those she loves like a bristling barbed wire. And she seems to understand in a way that I am just beginning to that it is all right to erect a boundary around yourself, even as you care for others.

Jason's brown eyes fill with tears and his mouth tightens and slips to one side in an attempt to muscle through emotion. Megan moves to my brother and wraps her arms around him, leaning her head against his arm. Barely reaching his shoulder, she stands strong as Jason seems to sag a bit. He runs a length of her hair through his fingers the same way he still "silkies" the satiny edge of a blanket.

"We can figure this out," Jason says after a moment. His voice is even and soft.

I am not used to seeing my brother with his defenses down. He is doing all he can to react to this in a measured way. It takes a tremendous amount of effort.

After my parents divorced and Dad married La, I stayed with them and Jason lived with my mom and we didn't see each other that much. When he was a sophomore and I was a senior in high school, he wore thrift-store bowling shirts, old tuxedos, and creaking leather oxfords, while I played it safe in pastel shaker knit sweaters from The Limited and Guess jeans with zippers at the ankle. While I stuck with my few girl friends and fellow theater geeks, Jason's circle of friends expanded to include the E Hall Freaks and the B Hall Brains and everyone in between. It bugged me that in just over a year he'd made a bigger social splash in school than I ever would.

It wasn't until I was at Northwestern and he spent a year at the Art Institute in Chicago that we got to know each other on neutral territory. I remember his visits to my apartment in the suburbs and how nice it was to be able to make him dinner, pour him a glass of milk, and give him fare for the train home.

Jason moved home to Albuquerque after two years in Chicago and finished up his art degree at UNM, where he met Megan. As a tattoo artist, he plies his trade on cops and gangbangers and housewives from gated communities. Somehow he is able to talk to everyone.

Jason and I join hands and head out into the driveway. Dad has stopped gluing pennies and sits on the wooden stump where in winter we split kindling for the wood stove. As we approach, he holds his hand up to shelter his eyes against the sun.

"So, the cavalry arrives," he says. "What's on your minds, children?"

Jason and I hunker down on either side of Dad. We look across at each other, trying to decide who's going to start this thing off.

"You know how you want everything to be ready when you go out on the road?" Jason starts slowly. "You need your brushes, your paints, and your ladders in the truck?"

"What are you getting at, Junior?" Dad asks.

"You wouldn't go on the road without taking the truck over to the mechanic for a checkup," I say. I look at Jason. I'm not sure this metaphor is working.

"You guys are trying to get me to the doctor," Dad says. "Carla put you up to this, didn't she?"

"We're worried too," I say. "We just want to make sure you're okay."

"I'm fine," Dad says. "I'm old, I'm tired, I'm a little crusty, but I'm fine."

"I'd appreciate if you'd do this for me." Jason's voice is gentle. "I'm getting married. I've got to have everything lined up, Dad. I need to know you're healthy."

Dad takes a long look at Jason and reaches an arm around his shoulder. "This is important to you? You're really serious."

"Getting married is serious business," Jason says.

"And what have you got to say here, Daughter?" Dad asks.

"I think we should get you checked out. Maybe we could go together while I'm home."

"Well, then, okay," Dad says.

We shake on it. Jason and I stand and help Dad to his feet.

"I love you," I say.

"I'm mighty fond of you too," Dad returns.

It is an old routine and we both laugh.

Jason sighs with relief. "Well, I could use a beer."

"Now that's where we're all in agreement," Dad says.

The Weeping Women * *April 1997*

SUNLIGHT POURS THROUGH THE WINDOWS of the waiting area of the Lovelace clinic. Dad and La and I fidget in the coral-colored chairs as we wait for our name to be called.

"This is taking too long," Dad says. "What do you say we hit the road?"

"Come on, honey," La cajoles, resting her hand on Dad's knee. "You promised."

"You women and your promises," Dad says.

I am scared and I think Dad is too. Across from us a young man sits next to a tiny old woman whose white hair stands out in wisps around her head like clouds on a windy day. She looks confused and moves her mouth as though she is feeling words against her teeth, trying to sort them with her tongue. I look at Dad. He's wearing a clean western shirt and his reddish hair is neatly combed. He is thinner than usual, but otherwise, he looks vital and alive in a way that this old woman does not. At fifty-eight, he's got years before he starts to fade at the edges like this. Doesn't he?

When our name is finally called, La and I and Dad squeeze into a small examination room. The doctor is young and wears his blond hair in a sort of shag. He's wearing a cream pullover sweater with a zipper at the neck and lime green suede loafers. He is not the right fit for Dad, who can't seem to stop his eyes from rolling back in his head whenever the doctor turns away from him. Dad points out the doctor's shoes and makes a face.

La and I talk a lot and Dad talks very little. I tell about the time a couple of nights ago when we stopped at a row of news boxes and Dad jumped out of the truck to get the evening paper. He returned with an armful of newsprint that included the *Autobuyer*, a Spanish language publication, and several real estate pamphlets. When we pointed out his mistake, he got angry and wondered why we'd want to read so much bad news anyway. The doctor nods and writes notes in a careful block print. La jumps in to answer nearly every question and eventually the doctor asks her to let Dad answer on his own. He asks Dad to repeat a list of words and to tell him today's date. Dad remembers four out of five of the words, but doesn't know the month or day.

"We can't rule out Alzheimer's," the doctor says. "But we're going to want some more tests." He explains that Dad will be tested for vitamin B6 deficiency and for lead poisoning. He adds that there's no way to make a definitive diagnosis of Alzheimer's without sampling brain tissue postmortem in a search for plaques and tangles. The plaques accumulate in the tissue, weighing it down, crushing the life out, and the tangles constrict blood flow until the brain shrivels. The memories are the first to go, the doctor tells us, followed by language and then, all bodily functions. "You literally forget to breathe," he says.

La and I both start to sob. Dad looks at us and at the doctor and for the moment decides to align himself with the doctor.

"Can you believe these weeping women?" he asks.

We are in the truck on the way back up to Tinkertown. La pushes her hair out of her eyes and squeezes Dad's knee.

"That guy was an asshole," Dad says. "What was he—twenty? What's a kid like that know about anything anyway?"

When I was about six, I burned my thumb on a candle at Pete's Mexican Fare, our local restaurant. I cried out and Dad dunked my whole hand into my water glass and picked me up and carried me out of the smoke and noise and into the quiet, cool night. He held me against his hip and looked me right in the eye.

"That's some burn you've got there," he said. "It makes me think of the time Campfire Sally got that big antler stuck in her thumb."

In the first of what would become a series of stories, Dad told how Campfire Sally (who happened to have long, brown hair just like mine) was out on a picnic with her red-bearded dad, Buckskin Joe, and somehow managed to get an elk antler stuck right in her thumb.

"It was the biggest splinter you'd ever seen," Dad continued. He told me that Campfire Sally screamed and cried just like I was doing, but eventually with strong pliers and good luck, Buckskin Joe was able to pull that antler right out, and she survived. "She did better than just survive," Dad said. "She had a great story to tell."

I wonder what kind of spin Buckskin Joe could put on plaques and tangles. Are they some kind of sand snakes, crawling up the bedpost in the night, entering through an ear and curling into the brain to nest and feed? Will he survive this? If he doesn't, who will tell the story?

The Diagnosis ✳ *February 13, 1998*

AT FIRST, IT LOOKS LIKE thyroid problems and a vitamin B deficiency are the reasons for Dad's forgetfulness. But eighteen months after that first doctor's appointment, the medication hasn't kept his words from disappearing.

One night I dream that I am walking through Dad's workshop. The floor is covered with a spongy layer of sawdust. Scrap two-by-fours are scattered at the base of the band saw, waiting to be thrown into the woodstove. There's no fire now and it's so cold, I can see my breath. The workshop smells of paint thinner, wood smoke, and the sweetness of WD-40, a lubricant Dad uses to keep the motors in the museum running. On the workbench are several small, wood-carved people. Using scraps from his old clothes, Dad has dressed the figures in tiny blue jeans and western shirts. He has painted boots on their feet. I pick up one of the figures and realize that it is a likeness of my father. He sports a well-trimmed, reddish beard, wears his customary Levis covered with splotches of paint and holds a tiny bottle of beer. I hold the figure for a moment and then, without thinking, I break off his head.

The next morning, La, calls me, crying. I'm at work, sitting in a cubicle in the middle of the writers' office of *The Tom Show*, a recently canceled ABC sitcom starring Tom Arnold. I put her on hold and run from my desk into my boss's office, closing the door behind me. When I pick up the phone again, I am crying too because I know what she is going to say.

After I hang up the phone, I sit for a long time watching the Universal Studio Tour buses troll up and down the street outside.

"Whatcha doin'? Taking over the show?"

My boss hunkers in the doorway of his office. He's built like a bear—a big, Irish bear. His eyebrows come together and the smirk slides off his face, replaced by a frown of concern.

"Are you crying?"

I nod and tell him about Dad.

"There's a lot I'd like to forget," he says. When he doesn't get a laugh, he pats his pocket. "Smokes?"

I nod and together we go downstairs to the front steps. He shakes out a couple of cigarettes, and when I put mine between my lips, he leans over with his huge hands cupped around the lighter. I take a deep breath and fill my lungs. My head spins. A tour bus passes and we wave automatically, making ourselves part of today's attraction.

"Is there anything I can do?" he asks.

I squint up at him. I want to say, "You can stop asking me to get your coffee. You can stop telling me I'm so smart. You can hire me as a writer instead of an assistant." Instead, I shrug.

"Take off early," he says. "It's dead here and you deserve a rest."

I call my mom from the car. I want to tell her about Dad's diagnosis so she doesn't hear it from someone else. Though they divorced when I was twelve, her feelings will be hurt if she's left out of this situation. After my parents' split, I elected to live with my dad, but I felt keenly responsible for making sure information was evenly shared with both of my parents. This was sometimes as easy as passing on a mimeographed flyer for a band concert or a school play; at other times, keeping things fair was a bit harder to manage.

When I got my first period, I shouted to La for help. She rushed into the bathroom and pulled out a wealth of supplies she'd purchased in advance. She showed me how to use the pads, gave me a quick pitch on the efficiency and comfort of tampons, and fled the bathroom. When I emerged, she'd filled a hot water bottle and made me a cup of tea.

A day later, I was visiting my mom's house, trying to figure out how to announce that I'd hit this big feminine milestone without her around. I couldn't think of a way to tell her without making her feel left out, so I went into the bathroom, took out the pad, carefully hid it in the bathroom trash and gave a big shout. Mom rushed to my side, hugged me, cried, and pulled out a box of pads she'd been keeping on hand for this very occasion. At dinner that night she toasted my entry into womanhood and my brother rolled his eyes and readjusted the headphones on his Walkman.

My mom is out. Her answering machine tells me to have "a blessed day."
I'm a teensy bit grateful that I can keep this terrible news to myself for just
a bit longer. I punch in my dad's number and continue to drive.

"Hey, kid," he says.

"Hey. La told me," I say. "How do you feel?"

"Listen," he says. "Everything will be all right. Everything will be fine."

He tells me he is reading a book about the brain. He tells me that the
doctors don't know everything even though they think they do. He says he
isn't worried. We've gotten through a lot of stuff. We'll get through this too.

"Can you believe I'm talking to you on a cell phone?" I say. "I'm just
leaving Universal Studios. It's pretty ridiculous."

"You're the Hollywood Kid," he says.

"I don't know," I say.

Dad is quiet, but I don't want to hang up. I want him to keep talking. I
want to keep the phone pressed to my ear, listening, listening.

"I love you," I say.

"I'm mighty fond of you too," he replies.

I try to laugh. The exchange takes on a new weight. How long will he
continue to remember this joke? What will I say when he forgets?

Unique and Special * *February 1998*

ON MONDAY MORNING, I drive to the Alzheimer's Association and pick up a copy of *The 36-Hour Day*. The cheery blue and orange cover boasts that the book has helped half a million families. I take the damn thing to Griffith Park and stretch out on a blanket in the sun. I need to be close to grass and the sound of children laughing.

In the first chapter I learn that the word *dementia* comes from two Latin words meaning *away* and *mind*. The book tries to console me with the fact that "many brilliant and famous people have suffered from dementing illnesses" and reminds me that the person with dementia is still a "unique and special human being."

After reading chapter 1, I throw the book down and turn over on my back to stare at the sky. The sun feels good on my skin. Dad loves the sun. He likes to cover himself with Hawaiian Tropic tanning oil and laze about in the backyard wearing nothing but a pair of teensy leopard briefs. He's painted numerous signs and nailed them around the property. One of them reads, "Don't be rude, get nude," while another warns, "Naked sunbathing beyond this point." I grew up knowing that when I saw the curve of his beer belly rising above the edge of the hammock, I'd better stop and shout "hello" just in case he'd shed his jungle pants. Eventually, he built himself a round enclosure with a six-foot fence and a gated entrance where he could lie in repose, nude and unbothered.

I sit up and grab the book again. I read about how dangerous a normal household can become for a person with dementia. I read about the loss of independence, temper tantrums, choking, and tube feeding. I read about incontinence and adult diapers and seizures. When I get to a section titled in capital letters, "DEATH OF THE IMPAIRED PERSON," I am less than halfway through the book. The sun has traveled across the sky and people around me are folding up their blankets and dousing their barbecue fires.

In 1975, when I was six years old, it dawned on me for the first time that my father was going to die. I was watching a local science show hosted by Albuquerque mom Kathleen McVicker. A housefly, she said, lives for a couple of days. A dog or cat lives for up to twenty years. A human can expect to spend somewhere around eighty years on the planet. A tortoise outlives us all with a lifespan of more than one hundred years. Little cartoon images accompanied this information. The human was represented by a bearded man wearing a fringed vest and platform shoes. That man could have been my father.

"I'm not going to die," Dad said. "I'm thirty-five years old. I'm not going anywhere. I promise." He held me tight before beginning to tickle my sides with his thick, round fingers. "Don't smile," he teased.

"Quit it," I said and wriggled in his grasp. I knitted my brows and tried to frown.

"That's right, I don't want to see any laughing. This is serious business here." He continued to tickle me until, still wet-faced from my tears, I laughed.

"See, it's fine," Dad said. "Nobody is dying. I'm staying right here with you."

Back in my apartment, I call Dad.

"What's it like?" I ask.

"What's what like?"

"How does it feel when you forget?"

"It's like I'm setting a table," he says. "Everything is all laid out. The plates, the glasses, the napkins. The silverware is in the right place. It looks great. I'm just about finished. And then, something happens—I'm not even sure what—but it all starts to slide. At first, I try to put things back, but pretty soon, I don't know where they go. And then, I don't even know what they are."

I am silent for a moment.

"The other night," he says, "I went to the drawer in the kitchen for a knife and once I opened the drawer, I just stood there thinking 'knife' but I didn't know what to pick up."

"Are you scared?" I ask.

"Hell, yes," he says.

Moving Grandma West * *March 1998*

SEEN FROM THE AIR, Aberdeen, South Dakota, is flat in all directions. In February the land looks like the inside of an old freezer, dull beneath a layer of frost. Train tracks crisscross the city. Small wood-frame and brick houses line the streets. Dark tree branches claw the sky. As we make our descent, I think about the last time I spoke to my grandmother. "Alzheimer's is about the worst thing you can have," she said through tears. "Ross needs me." Though she's spent her entire life in Aberdeen, Gran has decided to move to New Mexico to look after her only child.

As La and I step out of the tiny airport, our breath billows up in frigid clouds. It is nine degrees.

"Holy shit," La says.

When we arrive at Grandma's apartment the door is slightly ajar. We enter and she crosses to me quickly and hugs me fast, as though she is afraid I will run.

"Are you hungry?" she asks. And then, "Sit a while. Are you warm enough?"

She rubs my arms to warm me. I follow her to the sofa, where she sits, her hands methodically smoothing the rust-colored velour upholstery. Except for the stack of white packing boxes in the corner, almost everything else in the apartment is brown. Brown sofa, brown chairs, brown tables. Brown particleboard bookshelves. The shag carpet is a mix of brown and rust—"high-lo" it's called.

It is at least ninety degrees in Grandma's apartment. Though I have stripped off a couple of layers, I can feel sweat prickle under my arms and bra straps. Grandma, in her turtleneck, blouse, and sweatshirt, seems impervious to the heat, but from deep within her layers of polyester comes a slight fruity rot, like bananas left too long in the sun.

We go to dinner at a place called The Flame, which has been serving big steaks and baked potatoes since my dad was a rebellious teen. Like most things in this town, it hugs the railroad tracks. I slide into the red Naugahyde booth and take in the dark wood walls. While our waitress lights the candle in the round, red tabletop votive, she informs us that we can get walleye, which is the South Dakota state fish. Grandma orders a chicken sandwich, while Carla and I opt for steaks and baked potatoes. When our wine arrives, La ignores Grandma's disapproving look and holds her glass up in a toast.

"You know," she says, "I never eat red meat, but it just seems sort of . . . I don't know . . . appropriate."

"Yep," I say. "To meat."

"I never had but one boyfriend," Grandma says.

La and I look at each other in surprise. We are not used to Grandma's sudden and random bursts of information. Sometimes she seems to blurt out the answer to a question we have not asked.

"That was Grandpa, right?" I say.

"I made him wait four years before we were married," she says.

"Wow," we say.

When I was ten, I spent my birthday money on a book of poetry by Shel Silverstein. I included some carefully copied poems in my thank-you note to Grandma and she wrote back that while she didn't read much poetry, Grandpa had written some poems for her when they were courting. I wonder how many poems he wrote in those four years, what they were about, and where they are now.

"Everyone thought they'd see me pregnant before they'd see me married," Grandma says. "But I wasn't."

She gives a snort of satisfaction before tucking into her chicken sandwich. *Was it luck or lack of trying?* I wonder. I share a quick smile with La before turning my attention to my steak.

Back at the apartment, Grandma pushes my hands away and climbs out of the car on her own. The sidewalk has grown icier, and I walk behind her, ready to catch her if she falls. In her coat, she is a small aqua rectangle, her head wrapped in a scarf. Just before we reach the front steps, she wobbles a bit and I am right there, holding her elbow. She shakes me off again and reaches into her pocket, her mittened hand resurfacing with a bright pink, plastic spiral key chain. She slips the spiral around her wrist and climbs the stairs.

"I am not feeble," she says. "Don't you two forget that."

Grandma has decided that La and I will take her bed and she will sleep on the sofa. When we protest, she explains that the sofa folds out, but then refuses to let us unfold it. She switches off the lights in the living room, but sits upright, waiting for La and me to get settled. I do not know if she sleeps. I do not know if she ever lies down.

La and I negotiate the bedroom. There is a large crucifix above the bed, a porcelain figure of the Virgin on the dresser, a color print of Jesus Christ on the opposite wall. We climb into Grandma's bed, both of us trying to leave the other as much space as possible. I've brought a book to read, but all I can think about is Dad.

"How is he?" I ask. La can't even get through a sentence in reply before I start to cry.

La cries too. We talk of money and of care and somewhere in the middle of it, I realize that the enormous love I have for my father is more than matched by La's love for her husband. Eventually, we are cried out. I sleep until my legs grow numb from hanging off the edge of the small bed and I wake up to darkness and the sound of the ticking clock, my heat-flushed cheeks still damp to the touch.

Dishwater pale, the morning comes not a minute too soon. We are up and about, ready to go. We've got to clear out all the bank accounts, close the safety deposit box and deal with the bonds that Grandma bought from a man who "comes some Tuesdays." Grandma carries all her important papers in a plastic folder tucked inside a yellow canvas bag bearing a picture of a smiling frog. She will remark a number of times during this day, "It's my money. You don't get none of it. You got your own."

After the bank, we drive out to the cemetery to visit Grandpa's grave. When her time comes, Grandma will be buried right next to him in a plot that has been paid off for years. For my grandparents, death is the only real reason to splurge. At Grandma's direction, we trudge into the "Garden of Resurrection" and soon realize that flat grave markers are no help when covered by six inches of snow. Where is Grandpa? Gran thinks he's about six feet back, over by a small tree, to the left . . . no, the right. We scrape snow off the ground with our feet and find Brown, Drake, and Peterson, but no Ward. "Are you sure?" we ask. "I should know where my own husband is," she sniffs. And so we continue. We shuffle in circles radiating out from the small tree. Eventually, all the snow in the Garden of Resurrection is turned over and Grandpa is still lost. Grandma has stopped searching and stands with her back to me, staring off at the horizon.

La and I seek help in the small brick cemetery office. The far wall of the front room is covered with sheets and sheets of graph paper. Penciled names in a smudged and spidery hand make up a map of the entire yard. Bits of yellowing tape are scattered across the surface as shiny as fingernails. We peer at the map and see that, there, directly across from the Garden of Resurrection, is Ward, Everett. To Grandma's credit, there is a small tree nearby and he is about six feet from the road.

We head back out to Grandma. After we convince her to cross to the other side, we find Grandpa in a matter of moments. We pose for a photo next to the brass plaque. Grandma holds tight to my arm, but she does not speak. As soon as the shutter snaps, she moves toward the car without a backward glance.

The light is turning dusky blue and the wind has picked up. We realize we are starving. Tonight, we head to a place called The Refuge, where we are ushered into a large room with a vaulted ceiling.

"Look up," La says. And when I do, I am eye to glass eye with a forest full of critters. Fish, geese, and a snarling fox share shelf space with raccoons and a family of pheasants. A doe head gazes liquidly at a couple of bison heads across the way.

"Some refuge, huh?" La says.

The food is good and the wine seeps into us, thawing our bones and relaxing our shoulders. I wish that Dad were with us. La and I call him nightly, checking in on him, so much more aware that he is alone. He thanks me for coming to Aberdeen in his place. I look across the table at my wiry, blonde stepmother and at Gran in her bright pink sweater, her glasses glittering on her nose. The troops are gathering. Here, in Aberdeen, South Dakota, surrounded by a taxidermy wilderness, three generations of women are taking the first steps toward acceptance.

Back in the apartment, I settle into a chair with a cup of tea, trying to thaw a bit.

"What'll you charge me to wash my hair?" Grandma says.

"Nothing," I say. "It's on the house."

"We'd better do it quick before you change your mind," she says and disappears into the kitchen.

Moments later, she reappears, stripped down to a white brassiere with a towel over her shoulders. She hands me a bottle of shampoo. "Are you ready?"

Grandma leans over the sink and I let the tap water flatten her wiry little curls. This is the first time I have seen the smooth, white skin of her back, the soft dimples in her shoulders and the downy hollow at the base of her neck. This is a place I like to be kissed. Were my grandfather's lips ever pressed to this spot? Did his arms slide around her waist to pull her against him? Because my father exists I know this must have happened once. I want to think that it happened more than once. I want to think that there is something wild and restless in my grandmother. I want most of all, to see some trace of my passionate, rebellious father in this still and silent woman.

The next morning Grandma is silent and I am frightened for her because, next to the death of my grandfather, this move is the biggest change she has ever had to endure. As we wait for the movers, she wanders around the apartment, picking up odds and ends that have fallen somewhere between the packing boxes and the trashcan. She finds a brown plastic lid, a couple of miniature Hershey bars, and a roll of plastic wrap. She holds each of them for a moment before setting them down in a neat row on the countertop and retiring to the sofa.

"This couch is practically new," she says.

"That's why we're bringing it to New Mexico," La assures her.

The movers arrive. Two gawky twenty-somethings take orders from a heavily muscled black man with a wicked sense of humor. La and I drink in his banter and let it wash over us and the dryness of Aberdeen. My grandmother watches suspiciously as he scoops up her rocking chair and heads out the door.

"That's a pretty good job for a black," she says.

"Let's go pick up some lunch," La says. "Tanya will make sure everything gets in the truck."

Grandma puts her coat on and ties her scarf securely under her chin. "Well, all right," she says. "But I'm buying."

La nods and ushers Gran out the door. I watch from the window as La hovers around Gran, staying close, but never touching the bunched figure in the bright blue coat.

We spend our last night in Aberdeen with my father's cousin, Dick, and his wife, Ann. Dick is a wiry, cheerful man with graying hair and slightly bucked teeth.

"You could say I'm eccentric," he says. "Just like your dad."

"Now let them get settled," Ann says.

"Hey," Dick says, "You want to see me make fire from flint and steel? I'm a mountain man, you know."

In the living room, we watch as Dick places straw and a piece of carbon cloth in the fireplace. He takes a smooth bit of flint from a small leather pouch and begins to strike it with a piece of steel. Sparks fly and Dick blows hard, his cheeks puffing with the effort. The straw catches, then peters out. Dick blows harder, scattering ashes over the carpet.

"It's always like this," Ann says. "The minute I get this room clean, Dick's back in here with the flint and steel."

"Here we go," Dick shouts. And there, on the edge of the fireplace, a tiny flame licks at the straw and begins to brighten.

The next morning, Ann, in a sweatshirt that reads, "Life by the yard is hard, by the inch a cinch!" pulls a tray of muffins from the oven and pours coffee into brightly colored mugs. Grandma sits quietly, picking at her muffin while Dick loads the car.

At the airport Grandma clutches my hand, letting me support her for the first time in four days. Her lip trembles. She hugs Dick and Ann so tightly that I know she has realized she will never see them again. For the umpteenth time I wonder if this is right. She made the decision to leave, but I wonder if she knows what she's doing. As we walk to the plane, Grandma walks between us, reaching for our hands like a child.

In my seat, I watch as Aberdeen grows small below us. As we head west, Grandma claims she sees tiny men on the wing of the plane. She tells us that they're standing there, waving to her. She wonders how they can breathe. La gives Grandma's hand an extra squeeze and says, "They just can. They have no choice."

Have You Thought About Coming Home?
* *July 1998*

FOUR MONTHS LATER, icy Aberdeen is a distant memory. It's July and my apartment must be about a hundred degrees. Beyond the dusty screen door, the sun bathes my street in flat, bright light. La has been calling nearly every day.

"I don't want to stress you out," she says. "But have you thought about coming home?"

It's all I think about. David and I talk about it nonstop. My friends all weigh in. I ask the man at the post office as he's selling me stamps what he would do. I ask the guy who bags my groceries and the woman who cuts my hair.

Aside from David, there's not much to keep me in L.A. I'm out of work and waiting for my former boss to make up his mind and hire me as a writer. This boss is the most recent in a long line of older guys. They all have petite blonde wives and a dark sense of humor. I answer their phones and organize their files. I set up meetings and only occasionally pick up their dry cleaning or take their convertibles to the car wash. They think I'm fun to have around. They sometimes tell me I'm beautiful. They always tell me I'm smart. Too smart to work in television, they say. I've joined them for lunch, gone with them to pick out carpet, cars, and anniversary presents and sat next to them in the darkened rows of empty matinee movies. When I describe my job, I often say I'm a great date without any sex.

La tells me I'll have a real job if I come home. La's brother Fritz has recently married her best friend Mari, who runs a small ad agency. Fritz and Mari have sold their house to Jason and Megan because they are moving to the Bahamas to start a new life together. La has decided that she and Megan and I should take over the ad agency.

Though Megan is a terrific artist and I can write, we know nothing about running an ad agency. La is convinced it will be no problem. She's promised to manage our finances and let us take on all the creative stuff.

"This is happening for a reason," La says. "It's an opportunity we have to take."

Though La is sometimes an almost backbreaking realist, she is also the person who suggested I go on *Jeopardy* as a way of making ends meet while I was looking for my first job in Los Angeles.

I feel woefully underqualified, but I like the idea of running an agency. It sounds like a grown-up plan. At the very least, I might be able to make enough money to pay off my credit cards and start over. Recently, I went to the ATM to withdraw forty dollars and found that I had insufficient funds. After a few frantic phone calls, I realized that the last time I paid my bills, I had written a check to my Visa card for the balance in my checking account instead of the minimum balance owed. I was flat broke for a week and spent the entirety of my next paycheck on fees for overdrafts and returned checks. I imagine that as an executive of an ad agency, I will no longer have these kinds of problems. From this new stable vantage, I might be able to figure out what it is I really want to do.

One night, David is over. He wants to order a pizza, but I've got Nanci Griffith cranked up on the CD player and I'm all gloom and doom.

"Look," he says, "I don't want you to go, but you're driving us crazy here. You've got to figure this out."

I think I have already figured things out. Despite all the possibilities that Los Angeles holds for me, New Mexico is still the only place I can call home. My family are the people I love the best, and I am hardwired to be with them. I take a deep breath.

"I'm going home," I say.

David wraps his arms around me and we stand like this for a long time. I love him, but I don't feel like this is the right time for "happily ever after." Dad's illness has shaken my world so hard that the only way to put one foot in front of another is to make tracks for home. When the shaking stops, I only hope David is still here waiting.

The next six weeks are a blur. When I announce that I am moving home, everyone cries. La, my brother, my mother, my friends. Some people call me a "saint." It is oddly elating to so suddenly feel a sense of purpose. Everyone is impressed except my dad. He says, "But I thought you lived in Los Angeles." He says, "You're coming home? For how long?" He says, "Life in L.A. isn't exciting enough? You've got to move in with the geezer?"

The doctors give Dad five years to live. Early onset Alzheimer's moves fast, slashing and burning its way through the brain. Five years. It is impossible for me to think about this, and so I assume I am going to New Mexico forever.

Three days before I go, my brother, Jason, flies out to help me finish packing and keep me company on the drive home. I am so glad to see him my heart feels like it will jump straight out of my chest. An hour later, I watch him tip a kitchen drawer full of silverware into a box filled with bathroom towels

"You're mixing rooms," I say.

"I'm packing," he says. "It's all going to the same place. Sort it out later." He picks up the box and adds it to the pile in the living room. I trail along after him, holding a Sharpie.

"Let me at least label it," I say. "I need to know where things are. I need to know what's what."

"Chill out, Tanya," he says. "It's not a big deal."

"Not to you," I say.

"Hey," he says. "I'm trying to help."

I let out a sob. Jason hugs me fast and tight as though he might be able to stop the flow of tears with the pressure of his arms around my body. When I look up at him, he smiles and then he makes the strange, sad face of a very old, deaf, and blind poodle we saw once when we were kids. Whenever he makes this face, I can't help but laugh. Jason and I don't talk on the phone much. We don't keep up on the day-to-day details of each other's lives. But we can rely on a kind of short hand with each other that we don't share with anyone else. I am grateful for this connection. If, one day, I have a child of my own, I'll be sure to have another so that they can keep each other company when the going gets rough.

A while later, I am carefully wrapping my collection of antique creamers in newspaper while Jason clears off the shelf above the kitchen sink.

"Hey," he says. "Where did you get this?"

I turn to see that he is holding a small ivory carving.

"Dad gave it to me the last time I was home," I say.

"Well, that sure is funny," Jason says. "Did he tell you what it was called?"

"It's a *netsuke*—Japanese ivory carving. He said he'd traded it for a sign," I say.

"He didn't trade it. I bought it for him in Hawaii," Jason says. "It's called 'The Man who Carried his Son in a Box.' In the story this guy saved his son by hiding him in a fishing box."

"You can have it back," I say.

"No, no, no," Jason says, turning away from me, so that it seems he's throwing his words over his shoulder. "You keep it. Dad gave it to you."

Jason won't meet my eyes. He is shrugging this off, but I can tell he's hurt.

"He doesn't remember things," I say, touching Jason on the arm.

"It wasn't that long ago," Jason says.

While Dad and I have always been close, his relationship with my brother has often been rocky. While Jason played soccer, my mom ran up and down the sideline, cheering until she was hoarse. Dad sat under a tree, his head bent over a sketchbook or a wood carving.

Dad built me a pink dollhouse with real shingles and working lights. We prowled bookstores together and made up silly songs in the truck.

"How's my best kid?" Dad would sometimes ask before quickly amending to "best daughter."

My brother will strip a greeting card of cash before tossing it into the trash and never gets attached to his possessions. Instead, he perpetually sells or trades his cars, guitars, and motorcycles, using each item as a step up to something else. He is not outwardly sentimental, but, like my dad, he has an eye for the perfect gift. That the ivory man was re-gifted to me is evidence of Dad's illness, but at this point, a lifetime of hurt feelings keeps Jason from seeing that.

The truck is packed and I leave tomorrow morning, but tonight we are celebrating. We've packed the house with friends. David's got his customary dishtowel thrown over his shoulder and is boiling water for lobsters. On his way out onto the porch to check the barbecue, he tops off my champagne and plants a kiss on my forehead. He is recreating my last birthday dinner, though I would be just as happy with the chicken over rice he served on our first date or the plate of spaghetti in red sauce he prepared while spouting lines from *The Godfather*, clad in a "wife beater" undershirt and suspenders.

My brother shucks corn and makes jokes. All the windows are open and the big fan is blowing cool night air. David's hands are rarely far from my body; his fingers in my hair, his head on my shoulder, his soft breath against the back of my neck.

We sit on the floor, cracking open lobsters with a pair of pliers and sucking the sweet flesh from the shell. There is ice cream for dessert and sweet, grilled plums. And a flurry of hugs and kisses when everyone leaves.

David and I make a bed for my brother on the couch. We check the lock on the truck and lay out my clothes for the morning. We kiss and kiss and cry a little more and then we are asleep, wrapped in each other's warmth, breathing in the same cool night air.

In the morning, I hold David's face between my palms and kiss him on the mouth. Early on, before I mustered up the courage to tell him I loved him, I used to say instead, "I really, really like you." He would smile because he knew what I meant and then he would tell me he "really, really liked" me too. I wipe away his tears and mine and he says, "Okay, now, I think you just have to go."

I swallow a huge sob and follow him down the stairs to the street. My brother is behind the wheel of the big truck. My small gray Honda is hooked on the back.

"I'll see you soon," I say.

"Just over three weeks," David says. "I'm already counting the days."

I give him one last kiss and jump into the truck and settle Wallace on my lap. Jason guns the engine and we pull away. That big sob bursts out of me and I turn around to see David. He is waving and waving, and then we round a corner and he is gone.

One Thing and Another * *August 1998*

IT IS NEARLY THREE in the morning when I roll down the driveway of Tinkertown. My headlights illuminate the green and brown bottle walls and pitched roofline of the museum. Stars pour out across the sky like sequins spilled from a jar. I snap a leash on Wallace before stumbling through the dark to the door of the house. As I fumble with the latch, I think of Jason. When I dropped him at his house in Albuquerque, an hour ago, the lights were on and Megan appeared on the doorstep in her robe. I think of how nice it must have been for him to come home to someone. I know that just across the driveway, Dad and La sleep curled together in the cottage. I let my exhaustion push aside my loneliness and open the door. Once inside, even with all the lights out, my feet know their way. In my old room, I pull off my clothes and curl into bed. In seconds, I am asleep.

A few hours later, just after seven a.m., La bounds into my room.

"It's time to get up," she says. "We've got to get that truck unloaded."

I sit up and rub my eyes. I look at the clock and look at La. "It's pretty early," I say. "I didn't even get in until after three . . ."

"We don't have room for the truck in the driveway. I can take you to town and we can return the truck and drive back together. I've got your dad started on the unloading."

La turns to go and I stare after her for a moment, waiting for this to sink in. Yesterday's long, hot drive across the desert with Jason seems as unreal as Dorothy's trip to Oz. I am home. And home is a working museum.

Suddenly, I hear a series of thumps followed by a crash. I jump out of bed, throw on my clothes from the day before, and swing open the screen door. Wallace races across the yard, stops for a quick furious roll in the dust, and then is off again, free and happy.

In the driveway, Dad is standing in the back of the truck, rubbing his head. My filing cabinet is sitting at an awkward angle on the ground.

"What happened?" I ask.

"Well, one thing and another," Dad says.

"That was too heavy to unload by yourself," I say. "We loaded one drawer at a time."

"Well, now, don't get all bent out of shape," Dad says.

"But why didn't you wait?"

"I thought I could just ease it off," Dad says.

"Well, you couldn't," I say. "And now it's wrecked." I am barely awake and already my things are being tossed around.

"What's going on?" La says, stomping down from Hannah the horse's corral with Dad's dog springing along at her heels. The lithe white dog— part terrier, part whippet—was a stray when La brought him home. Dad promptly christened him "Radar" because of his huge ears. Radar stops and narrows his dark eyes when he sees Wallace. The two dogs give each other a quick sniff before zooming together back up the hill. Wallace is already covered with a fine layer of red dust and looks happier than he has in a long time.

"Dad broke my filing cabinet," I say.

"Well, let's just get everything out and worry about it later," she says. She grabs a box and hands it to Dad and he starts off toward the cottage.

"No, honey," La shouts, "in the old house." I watch Dad waver for a moment in the driveway, before shifting direction and heading through the blue wooden door. Dad doesn't seem to understand what is happening. As I watch all my boxes make their way out of the truck, I wonder why I was so careful with the Sharpie. I wonder why I didn't let Jason dump the contents of every box straight into the trash bin.

When the truck is empty we all climb in and make the trip back down the hill, through the canyon and into Albuquerque. La tells me that tomorrow morning we'll have to take photos for the advertising agency press release. She's arranged for me to get a Costco card and made an appointment at the DMV so I can change my plates and get a New Mexico driver's license. She tells me the museum gates have to be opened by nine and closed at a quarter to six unless someone shows up. She tells me that Mari and Megan are getting the office ready and I can go down there in the next couple of days to train before Mari leaves. Dad doesn't say a word. At the rental truck place, we unhook my Honda and turn in the truck. We pile back into my car and head back up to the mountains to get the gates open. With La's voice in my ear, I drive well over the speed limit through the canyon.

"This is one hot set of wheels," Dad says. "If I had a car like this, I'd just drive away as fast as I could."

The House Where I Grew Up   ✳   *September 1998*

I UNPACK MY THINGS into what we call "the Tinkertown house." The other house, across the driveway, where Dad and La live now is what we call "the cottage."

They have only lived in the cottage for about a year, but in that time, the Tinkertown house, which was given over entirely to the four Tinkertown cats, is dirty and stale from disuse.

When La and I first talked about my move home, she told me she was considering moving with Dad back into the Tinkertown house.

"He loves it there," she said. "I think he'll be more comfortable. You can have the cottage. I'll get everything ready."

Then she changed her mind.

"I know your dad would like to live there again," she said, "but I just don't think *I* can." She promised to deep clean the place and outlined plans to add a French door.

"It'll be like a suite," she said. "You'll have your own suite with a private garden."

It sounded okay to me. Everything we talked about sounded good (perhaps only because the reason we were talking about it was so bad). We planned that I would take charge of the family kitchen and at the time, I'd had these wonderful *Gourmet* magazine visions of the three of us sharing one carefully prepared meal after another. I would research foods that were good for the brain and fill Dad's stomach with omega-3s and fresh veggies and we would eat and talk and really enjoy being together.

Now, that I've actually arrived, things seem different. La did not get around to having the house cleaned. The corners are filled with dusty spider webs, balls of cat hair roll like tumbleweeds across the scuffed wood floors, and there is very little unused space. The big, cold closet off my bed-room has been functioning as a catchall since I graduated high school and is crammed with old toys, boxes of debate trophies, my christening gown, a clown suit Dad wore as a child, La's lavender wedding dress, Nancy Drew books, beaded Indian belts from souvenir shops, and a bright orange steamer trunk emblazoned with tigers and my name in Dad's best circus-style lettering. Though it's a huge walk-in closet, there's less than three square feet of clear floor space. On the wall above the rack where I squeeze in my blouses, Benjamin Franklin is quoted in Dad's loose, penciled cursive: "Beware any enterprise that requires new clothes."

Even the water here has a habit of accumulation. Minerals form a crust on the cat's water bowl, leave a visible layer of white along the edges of the brown linoleum in the kitchen, and rim the lip of each faucet in the house like frost.

I open cupboards and closets and find the years layered one on top of another. In the kitchen, I find a B. Kliban placemat scattered with black-and-white cats that I used in fifth grade. On top of that is a folded stack of linen napkins that belonged to La's grandmother. Nearby is an apron I remember my mother wearing when she frosted the birthday angel food cakes of my youth.

Scratch the purple paint that Dad rolled over the kitchen in a flash of passion for La and you come up with the lime green my mother painted. The room where Dad and Mom slept is the one that La turned into her pottery studio when she married my dad. She spent days spattering clay on the walls and floors of what was once my mother's room and slept with Dad on a foam mattress in the living room alcove. Eventually, they added a bathroom and laid down midnight blue carpet in the room that we called Dad's shop.

"Nothing but the best for my lady," Dad said, peeling off hundred-dollar bills to pay for the lavender drapes in the newly christened "love nest." But outside he continued to build, and eventually the boardwalk allowed visitors to peer into the windows of the bedroom and a new building cut off the view of the trees.

I drag the vacuum from room to room, sucking up spiders and webs and balls of cat hair the size of my fist. I crawl around on the kitchen floor and scrub the linoleum until my hands are stiff and red. Dad follows me. He sits in the big, black leather rocker in the kitchen or perches on the purple stool made from an old tractor seat, folds his hands over his stomach and watches.

"So you're here for a while?" he asks.

"A while," I say.

"What about Los Angeles? I'd sure as heck want to get back."

"I'm happy to be here," I say. "I want to be with you."

"Well, this is a great old house," he says. "I sure wish I was moving into this place, but she doesn't want that. She wants what she wants and the old fart just goes along for the ride."

Dad pulls a pen and folded piece of paper out of his shirt pocket and, using his knee as a desk, begins to sketch. The details of a nude woman reaching skyward come together quickly as though the memory of this particular image lives in his hand more than his head.

"You know," he says, "I have this vision of being in this house when the big one comes—you know the big bomb—kablooey. And me and my old lady, we'll be making love. And the heat of the blast will melt the glass bottles around us and we'll be captured just like those insects inside a piece of amber. That'd be pretty wild, right? That's the way I'd like to go."

I'm beginning to understand why La needed to stay in the cottage. Because the Tinkertown house is embedded at the center of the museum, it is possible to be getting dressed in my bedroom and turn while fastening my bra to see an RV spilling a load of tourists into the parking lot. When I sit on the back porch, I hear children running up the wooden ramp that leads to the doll collection and the rattle of quarters jangling into Otto the band organ. The machine takes what seems to be a deep breath before blasting out a march or a waltz at top volume.

La claims the cottage has more light. She says it's easier to clean. And I'm sure it is. But it's clean in other ways too. It bears little weight of the past. The cupboards and closets hold only what is necessary to move forward from one day to the next. I think in making a move to the cottage La is weaning herself from the memories in the old house. Despite her love for my dad, she is unwilling to be caught when the big one comes.

Opening the Museum * *September 1998*

NEARLY EVERY MORNING since my arrival, Dad and I open the museum together. This morning is no different. I snap open the first padlock and rattle the chain through the heart-shaped hole cut into the front gate. Behind it is a cement courtyard embedded with dozens of rusty horse-shoes. A sign above the wrought iron grate of the ticket window tells you that adult admission is $3. "Geezers and geezettes" get the senior rate of $2.50, and kids are a buck even.

The dogs run ahead, snapping and biting at each other's legs, and Dad follows through the low wooden gate, cut out and painted to resemble the head of a long-horned steer. It swings open with a creak and, once we are through, bangs hard against a rainbow-colored rubber ball. The real cow-bell around the steer's neck jangles.

"Well, what have we got here?" Dad says when we stop in front of the display we call "The Band."

He drops a quarter in the slot, and Rusty Wyer and the Turquoise Trail Riders play what the sign says is "music fer all occashuns." Dad carved the band members and dressed them in clothes he sewed from scraps of his own. The guitar player wears a pair of bright red canvas tennis shoes that in the '70s belonged to my baby cousin, Gabe. The beady-eyed fiddle player wears a long, fur coat and a broad brimmed hat. Lead singer Rusty Wyer is decked out in a purple cowboy shirt with pearl snaps and looks out at the world through wire-rimmed glasses. Behind him stands a young girl in a polka-dot dress. Her eyes are glued on Rusty as her hands clap to the beat. The sign above her head tells us her name is Brancy and proclaims, "Rusty is my kind of man."

Today, we hear Patsy Montana rattle through "I Want to Be a Cowboy's Sweetheart." Just as abruptly as it starts, the tape clicks off, cutting Patsy's bright voice mid-word.

"Now ain't that something," Dad says. He seems genuinely impressed. Though he's never been short on self-congratulation, lately he seems mystified by all that he's done. I suppose you could say that the upside of Alzheimer's is that it makes every day seem like a surprise party. Dad seems hyperaware of the world and all its parts, stopping to admire a shiny beetle, a deep red rock, or just the feel of Radar's silky ears across his fingers.

We creak open the door to the shed that is home to Esmeralda, the life-sized Grandma fortuneteller whose chest rises and falls as her glass eyes scan the cards. Inside the museum are more quarter slots. Drop a coin in and a mummy emerges from a tomb, a steam engine whirs to life, or you test your strength by shaking hands with a metal figure of Uncle Sam. Whenever I grip the cold iron of Sam's gloved hand, bells ring, lights flash, and the arrow points to "twenty-eight-pound weakling."

Dad likes to go through the museum and empty the coin boxes into a big bucket. La says he's been squirreling away quarters somewhere. She wants to know where, but he won't tell her.

"It could be a lot of money," she says.

Wanting to please her, I ask Dad outright if he has a stash somewhere.

"Sure," he says. "Why wouldn't I rob the till. This is my place, right? I'm the mayor of Tinkertown. You need a little dough, Daughter?" He winks at me and takes me back into his workshop where he moves a couple of pieces of plywood to reveal an old suitcase. Inside the suitcase are dozens of rolls of quarters, dimes, and nickels.

"Here, get a load of this," he says. He puts my hand on the suitcase handle. "Just try to lift it. It's a mother, isn't it?"

"We should get the rest of the place open," I say.

"This is our secret, right?" Dad says. "She's always nosing around, but I don't want her to have it."

"Who?" I ask.

"Hoo-hoo," Dad says. He heads out of the workshop and down the path to the door of the western town where he stands, holding the lock in his hands.

"Do you need the combo?" I ask.

He clicks the numbers into place. "I know all this," he says. "I built this place."

We flick on the lights and Willie Nelson starts to sing. The album *The*

Red-Headed Stranger has been playing on a constant loop for as long as I can remember. Dad and I both sing, "It was the time of the preacher . . . ," drawing out the word "time" just as dramatically as old Willie himself. I can see Dad's reflection in the glass window as he pauses in front of the miniature country store. This was the first building he created, hammering together a frame of plywood and covering it with graying shingles salvaged from a desert shack.

He built the two-story Monarch Hotel next and carved the figure of Chantilly Freelance who has one suitor at the door and another about to climb out the window. A hand-lettered sign tells us that she's dedicated herself to a two-party system, "one in the morning and one at night." Downstairs, a man sits in a claw-foot tub, scrubbing his back.

"That was the hardest thing to work out," Dad tells me. "I had to get his arm to move without having a lot of visible wires . . . you can't wear clothes in the tub, right?"

He opens the door under the display and we duck down to take a look at the workings of Tinkertown—carefully bent wire coat hangers, pulleys made from strips cut from old inner tubes, and wooden thread spools along with dozens of sewing machine motors bring all the figures to life.

We stand up, brush off our knees, and he throws his arm around my shoulders as we stroll down past the blacksmith, the Lucky Nugget Saloon, and the soda shop known as Perry's Polar Pantry. I feel like I know the dusty streets of Tinkertown better than I know any city in the country. I think Dad would like to live in the little town. It's a perfect world for him. There's a huge toy store, all the women are pretty, the only restaurant serves Chinese food, and the circus is permanently set up just around the corner.

Years ago, when the western town was still in a trailer, we'd work the New Mexico State Fair, and Dad would keep me out of middle school for a day here and there to help run the show. In the morning, we'd lift the big wooden panels on the side of the trailer and set the support posts in place so that the panels formed a roof. We'd unroll a huge green canvas sidewall and clip it to eye hooks all along this roof so that people could walk around the trailer in the dark and look through the big glass windows at Dad's wood-carved village.

Once the show was up, I'd sit on a stool behind the plywood ticket booth, my hands in my change belt pockets, jingling the quarters through my fingers. On busy days, I'd take tickets and Dad would make change, peeling off ones and fives from the big wad he kept in the front pocket of his blue jeans. When the wad got too big to keep in his pocket, he'd head over to the beer tent to trade the small bills for larger ones and grab a plastic cup of Bud for himself and a Coke for me.

"You're in charge," he'd say. "Don't take any wooden nickels."

I'd sit up tall on my stool and wait for his return, scanning the crowd, hoping a friend from school would recognize me and see that I was more than just a chubby girl with a mouthful of braces and a bad perm. Eventually, I'd see Dad's gray felt top hat towering over the heads of the fairgoers. The hat along with a brightly colored velvet patchwork vest, his big silver Concho belt, and a Hopi eagle dancer bolo tie were part of what Dad called "flash" and came out of the closet any time he felt a need to be a part of the show.

We come out of the museum and into the gift shop and run smack into Maggie and Florence.

"Well, here they are, Fric and Frac," Florence says. She is a tiny woman in her sixties with a mouthful of big white teeth and a cap of hair that gets blonder with every trip to the beauty shop. She lives down the road with her husband, Demp, and has been working at Tinkertown for years.

"Like two peas in a pod," Maggie says with long, Bostonian vowels. She's tall and thin, with a prominent nose and a nimbus of pale apricot-colored hair. When Maggie's husband died a couple of years ago, Florence brought her up to Tinkertown for a job. They make a fine pair, sitting on the tall stools behind the cash register, their hands around twin thermoses of tea.

"Well, if it isn't Flossie and Maggie," Dad says. "Aren't you two a vision."

"I can see it in your eyes when you lie," Florence says.

Florence had been working at the museum for over a year when one day she asked Dad where he got the Jenny and he knew right away she was "with it." No one but a carny would call a carousel horse a Jenny. Turns out she used to run a cotton-candy booth, which in show vernacular is a "floss joint," so Dad always calls her Flossie.

"We knew there was something we liked about each other," she says about Dad.

"We're both so darned good-looking," Dad says.

"Well, there is that," Florence says dryly. "What are you getting into today?"

I tell her that I've got to get to the office. We've got a meeting with the Sandoval County folks to talk about a visitors' guide.

"Well, she sure has got you running, hon," Florence says. "I know this one here is glad as hell to have you at home."

"This one here?" Dad asks. "You mean the old geek with the brain disease?"

Florence's eyes fill up and she looks down, fiddling with the top to her thermos. "Well, Ross, you know it's nice to have your kid around. Even a blind person could see how happy you are about it."

"She's a good one," Dad says.

"For once we agree," Florence says.

On My Way to Work ∗ *September 1998*

I MAKE THE FORTY-FIVE MINUTE DRIVE to my new job, off the mountain into town. I am headed to the North Valley where Jason and Megan live in the house they bought from La's brother Fritz and his wife, Mari. Mari's business, once known as Anderson Advertising, has become Anderson/Ward Advertising and Design. It is run out of a large office just off the kitchen.

Right now we are in the middle of creating a brochure and logo for the Village of Corrales, which seems to be just a few old adobe buildings along the river. Because their brochure looked a bit thin with only the local attractions, we decide to add things "nearby," thus opening up the whole rest of the city and state. I realize quickly that the tourism business is just like the carnival business. Just as easily as the mild-mannered capybara can be billed as a "giant man-eating rat from the darkest heart of Madagascar," we can sell a town with one main street, no hotels, and two restaurants as a scenic and historic destination.

In a few short weeks, I have gone from being an out-of-work writers' assistant to being director of an ad agency. With my wallet full of business cards and a brand new Franklin Planner filled with deadlines, I have written radio ads for Cruel Girl jeans, rope bags, tack boxes, and something called a snaffle bit. I console myself with the fact that it's all "writing," but I feel like something is missing.

Dad calls me "the Hollywood Kid" and asks to be given a role on my television show. He tells me he'd like to ride in a helicopter with Tom Arnold. He says he'll do his own stunts. The probability of this actually happening is just slightly less than my selling a script and becoming a big-time writer. It was easier to be more optimistic in Los Angeles where hope vies with smog for air space. With every third person writing a screenplay or a spec script there is a kind of collective suspension of disbelief that keeps fingers pounding over keyboards. Here in New Mexico, out of context, screenwriting seems like spending grocery money on lottery tickets.

My job at the agency seems like a better bet, though despite La's faith in our skills, Megan and I continue to feel scared and uncertain. To cover the fact that we don't really know what we're doing, we've developed a system. I talk to clients on the phone and write down questions while Megan frantically flips through the glossary of terms in an old advertising textbook. When she nods, I assure the customer that we can carry out his request.

I learn that it is illegal to copy a map unless you have the rights to it, and so Megan spends a lot of her time drawing new maps for the brochures. We try to measure them against older maps to determine scale and make sure we are not leading visitors too far astray. I feel that I am drawing my own map these days too, holding it up to what I thought this move would be and then sitting back down to alter curves and erase expectations.

When the phone is silent, Megan and I tape up paint chips from the Martha Stewart line of paint at Kmart. We are eager to cover the muddy pink of the office walls. It's the dusty color you'd find in a cheap blush compact. We're thinking Willowware or Wicker or Seaglass. We want something light and airy and modern. Because neither Megan nor I has ever run an office, we are trying to create a perfect office setting. If we look like we can do it, then maybe we can.

I think of all the carnival dark rides Dad painted. Though you wouldn't know it from the outside, they are all basically the same: a big, empty box with a track running through it. It was Dad's job to create a promise of excitement that would convince the next bunch of local yokels to fork over a fist full of tickets for a ride through the dark. Each season, he covered the same old empty box with a new showfront. One year it was pirates or aliens and the next it might be cowboys or cannibals, each promising to deliver an adventure more spine-tingling, more hair-raising, more belly-churning than the last. It was only once you were inside, turning fast and loose in the blackness, that you realized it was an empty promise.

Nearly every morning, Megan and I sit on the front steps of her house, finish the pot of coffee, and smoke a cigarette. I've begun to look forward to this ritual. Any routine, no matter how small, gives me something to hang on to in the midst of so much upheaval.

"So, David's coming soon," Megan says, breathing a plume of smoke into the air. "You must be excited."

I'm about to shoot out of my skin with excitement, but instead I shrug. I feel the need to be calm about David around my family, and not let on how much I need him. I don't want to admit that there's a chance that something—someone—might be more important than my dad.

"I'm worried it'll be weird."

Megan's dog, Cecil, places a small, slobbery stick next to my foot and takes a step back. He lets out a long, high-pitched whine and looks up at me expectantly.

"Weird how?" Megan says.

"I don't know," I say, throwing the stick. The stocky little dog tears after it.

"You've done it now," Megan says. "He's never going to leave you alone." Sure enough, Cecil returns with the muddy nub of wood and sets to whining again.

"Go on, Cecil," Megan says. "Get." She squashes her cigarette out against the step before turning to me. "Your brother and I lived apart for a long time. I went back to Hawaii and then to San Francisco. But eventually, it worked out. It just took time. Try to take a deep breath. You know, just see what happens?"

I nod. She's right. I inhale the smells of dog slobber and smoke and damp earth. I fill my lungs with air and will myself to wait and see.

David's First Visit ∗ *September 1998*

THERE ARE VERY FEW PEOPLE in the Albuquerque airport this late at night and so I feel less self-conscious taking a minute to appreciate the carved wooden-beamed ceiling. This airport is dense with the history of expectation. My grandparents came and went, dressed in their good shoes for travel, my mother went to Europe and returned to this airport transformed, if only momentarily, by her experience. I ran alongside my college boyfriend through this airport all the way to the gate and then walked back alone and sobbing. This airport has witnessed all the comings and goings of my whole life. I slick on a layer of lip gloss, and then wipe it off with a tissue a moment later. I check the minutes on the cheap black clock that looks like it should hang over a teacher's desk, shove my hands into my pockets, and pace.

The minute I see David, all my nervousness evaporates. He hurries through the passenger gate and squeezes me tight. His leather coat creaks as I squeeze him back. His breath is warm against my neck and cheeks. We lean in to kiss and our noses bump together before our lips meet. His mouth is soft and his tongue tastes of peppermint. Suddenly aware of all the strangers around us, I pull away and tuck my arm through his.

In the parking lot, David throws his suitcase in the trunk and then climbs in next to me.

"I might need to make out a little more," he says.

I lean in and we kiss and kiss. His hand is on my leg, my breast, and in my hair. My breath comes quickly and I fight the urge to climb onto his lap and grind myself against him.

A car next to us flashes to life as arriving passengers load their luggage. I start to pull away from David.

"Let's get home," I say.

It is past midnight as we make the long drive through the canyon to Tinkertown with David's hand in my lap, my heart beating against my chest like a moth against a window.

We've slept for only a few hours and my cheeks are rubbed pink by the stubble on his jaw, my lips swollen from kisses. We are twined together, hovering just above sleep but awake enough to pull up the covers when the bedroom door swings open.

"Good morning," La says brightly. She's wearing jodhpurs and riding boots and carries her velvet riding helmet.

"Um, good morning," David says, his voice rising at the end of the word as though in question.

"I've got to take Hannah to a lesson, but your dad's up and in the bath and the museum is unlocked, you just have to turn on the lights. I should be back around noon, but it'd be great if you could throw a flake of alfalfa in for the other horse."

"Got it," I say. I am keenly aware of the thin sheet that covers our naked bodies.

Just as suddenly as she arrived, La is gone.

David and I wait until we hear the jangle of the front door latch and then we start laughing and can't stop.

"Holy shit," David says. "Is she always like that?"

Shortly after La married my dad, when I was around twelve, she gave me a book called *Changing Bodies, Changing Lives*.

"Read it," she said. "And come ask me if you have questions."

I learned where my breasts were coming from and that, someday, they could make milk for a baby. I learned about condoms and diaphragms and sexually transmitted diseases. I was a quick study and I learned a lot of things, but what I remember most about *Changing Bodies, Changing Lives* is that it taught me to masturbate. Before I read this book, I never, ever touched myself, but after I read this book and for a period of about six months, I touched myself nightly, sometimes two and three times. I kept very quiet throughout, holding the sheets above me so they wouldn't make a sound. Afterward, I tiptoed to the bathroom and washed my hands, feeling vaguely ashamed of the thrilling tingle I'd just experienced.

As I became more practiced, I concocted elaborate scenarios in my head. "Fuck me," I'd whisper through my retainer. "Fuck me, Han Solo,"

I'd moan, dreaming of my white knight, of my one true love, of someone, anyone, who could see the beauty hiding in my pudgy, shy, pubescent self.

Out in the museum, my old iron bed frame is now a fence. Dad calls it "the virgin bed." I wonder if, when she yanked open my bedroom door this morning, La was expecting to find that chubby girl with all the questions.

David and I are showered and dressed and drinking coffee when Dad finally gets out of the bathtub.

"Who's this?" Dad says.

"It's David," I say.

"Well, so it is," Dad says. "Big Dave. You moving here too?"

"Not yet, sir," David replies.

"Well, it's not so bad," Dad says, pulling up a chair at the table. He reaches into his shirt pocket for a ballpoint pen, flips open his sketchbook and starts to draw. A self-portrait quickly materializes followed by the quick outlines of a girl with my own bobbed hair. She points her finger at a callow-faced boy in overalls. Dad writes, "Yummy! Is that a David? Can I keep it?"

"Here you go, Daughter." He rips the page out of his sketchbook, saying cryptically, "More evidence."

I laugh with relief. I was unsure if Dad really recognized David or if he was confusing him with my previous boyfriend who was also named David. I can tell that David is stinging from being lumped in with my ex, but he musters a chuckle.

"You're not starting a collection, are you?" he says, wrapping an arm around my waist.

"It runs in the family," I tease, but then I give him a little bump with my hip and lock eyes for a minute so he knows for a fact that I'm done collecting.

It's nice to have David's company for a day of home duty, and Dad seems to relish having an extra audience member.

"You got a minute?" he asks again and again. Again and again we reply, "Yes."

He shows us dozens of his paintings and asks David to try to lift a bulky portfolio filled with his etchings.

"That's a mother, isn't it?" Dad says, beaming.

He shows us half-finished wood carvings and takes us to the circus room of the museum where we marvel at his model of the famous Two Hemispheres Bandwagon.

"Just something I've been working on lately," he says.

I know that he finished carving the wagon and all the members of the band who sit atop it years ago, but I keep quiet and let him bask in David's appreciation.

Dad shows David the way he can climb up the wall of the museum using the necks of the bottles as a ladder.

"That's amazing," David says. "Is it really okay?" he whispers to me.

I squeeze his arm and assure him that the bottles won't break.

We head down to the Burger Boy to grab green chile cheeseburgers from the old cowboy Dad always calls Green Chile Bill.

When our order comes, David pulls out his wallet, but Dad waves him away.

"Your cash is no good here, young fella," he says, pulling out his own wallet. "Lunch is on the Mayor of Tinkertown."

Dad pulls out a couple of bills and puts them on the counter.

"That oughta cover it," he says.

I look up at the cashier and then at David. He grabs the tray.

"Let the young fella do the heavy lifting. Lead the way, sir."

Dad gestures for David to take the lead and falls in behind him, high-stepping like he's suddenly in a marching band. I'm impressed by the easy way David steps in to help. I take a quick moment to count the crumpled singles, before dipping into my pocket to add another ten.

Green Chile Bill smiles at me. "Shoot," he says. "He's the mayor, right? Your dad can eat for free."

At the end of our first day, we gather in the cottage getting ready for dinner. La waits for a stick of butter to melt in a small cast-iron skillet before throwing in a handful of chopped garlic. She coats each slice of bread before tossing it into foil to be heated in the oven. David leans against the counter with a beer, while I make salad dressing. While we work, La asks after family. She wonders how his writing is going. This is only the second time she has met David and I am happy that she has held onto so much information about his life. She remembers his brother recently graduated from college and wonders what his father is doing in his retirement.

"Pop's got all these ideas," David says. "He wants to work retail, mostly because he'd like to use a cash register, and at some point he wants to run a meat slicer."

"Like in a deli?" La asks.

"It's just something he wants to do," David says.

"I don't see why he shouldn't," La says.

I realize that Alzheimer's has forced my dad into a kind of retirement.

He doesn't paint signs anymore, but he's still drawing and carving and his life here at Tinkertown isn't so very different from the one he's always had.

"Chuckwagon's on," my dad says, sauntering in from outside wearing only a small pair of leopard-print briefs. David's eyes widen, taking in my dad's beer belly and the lizard tattoos on his chest. Dad pulls up a chair at the kitchen table and stretches out one long, pale leg to admire his toes.

"What do you think?" he asks. He's painted his toenails a deep turquoise.

"Is that enamel paint, honey?" La asks.

"Sure is," Dad says. "Sherwin-Williams. Cover the earth."

After dinner, David washes dishes and I dry.

"So," he says, "your dad has really slim hips."

"That's your take away?" I ask, laughing.

"Trust me, I'm taking away more than that," he says with a smile. "I'll bill you for my therapy later."

"Hey, I've got a great idea," La says. "You guys should sleep outside tonight. It's a full moon. It'll be gorgeous."

"Wow," David says.

"I'll get the sleeping bags," La says over her shoulder as she heads out to the storage shed.

"You want to?" David asks.

"If you do," I say.

"Here we go," La says, returning with an armful of slick fabric. "You can even zip them together if you want."

"Oh, I want," David says into my ear.

On the second day, when the evening trip to the airport looms over us, we sit in an old Ferris wheel seat on the back porch in the sun. David opens pistachios and drops their shells into a ceramic mug. We don't talk much. I hold in my questions about the future and let my shoulders relax. I remind myself to be aware of the warmth of David's leg beneath mine, the smell of juniper in the air, and the hint of chill just beyond the sun that whispers of autumn.

If this were a Sunday in Los Angeles, we'd most likely have spent the day in bed reading the paper and drinking coffee. We might have taken a hike up through Griffith Park or walked down the street to the Tam O'Shanter for a beer and a turkey sandwich. Our responsibilities began and ended with the workweek. I don't feel that kind of liberty here. There is no moment at which I don't expect La or Dad to walk into my room and ask for something.

The trip to the airport is terrible. I can barely keep my voice from shaking. On the way from the parking lot to the terminal, we hold hands and lean against each other.

"I'll be back in less than a month," David says. "You better buy stock in Southwest Airlines."

"I'd rather buy plane tickets to Los Angeles," I say.

At the gate, he hugs me one more time and I kiss him hard on the mouth, trying to hold back my tears. With just a taste of his company I realize not just how lonely I've been these last few weeks, but how lonely I have been for him. I want to keep David in my life. For the first time, I realize how much work I will have to do to make that happen.

Fireworks * *September 1998*

THE NEXT EVENING, I return home from work to find Dad and La standing at the counter eating microwave burritos and popcorn.

"I was going to make fish tacos," I say.

"Well, you're late and we were getting hungry," La says.

"It's a long drive," I say. I feel angrier than seems reasonable.

"Maybe this whole dinner thing isn't going to work out," La says.

There's a beautiful piece of fish in the refrigerator along with fresh salsa I made this morning. I miss David. I feel like coming home was a huge mistake.

"It'll take just a minute to put dinner together."

"We're eating," La says.

"You do everything so fast," I shout. "Why can't you take time to enjoy things? Why can't you wait twenty minutes for a decent meal? Doesn't it matter to you?"

"Not the way it seems to matter to you," La says.

I let the screen door slam behind me and head across the driveway to the old house. I try not to think of the confused look on Dad's face. We shouldn't be yelling like this in front of him.

In the purple kitchen, I put water on to boil and get out pasta, sun-dried tomatoes, and some fresh goat cheese I bought at the farmers' market. I open a bottle of good wine I've hidden in the cupboard, pour some into a water glass, and take a couple of big swigs as I chop garlic. I drizzle olive oil into a pan, let it warm, and then add the garlic. There is no greater comfort than the aroma of garlic cooking in olive oil. I feel my shoulders begin to relax as this smell blankets the kitchen.

I am thankful that I unpacked my kitchen things. Most everything else is stored away, but my pots and pans hang from the rack and my wooden spoons and rubber spatulas are in a pitcher on the counter. An enormous steel fish poacher sits on a low shelf along with a cast-iron Dutch oven and various covered casserole dishes. My pots and pans are the only tangible evidence that I had a home of my own.

I am sitting at the table finishing the last of my pasta when I hear the front door open and close gently. I can tell by the even rhythm of the footsteps that it's my dad. He comes down the steps and sits across from me.

"Hey, kid," he says.

"Hey."

"That was some fireworks."

"Yeah. I'm sorry about that."

"You guys gonna fight like that all the time?"

"I hope not," I say.

He takes the edge of the red cotton tablecloth and rolls it all the way up to the edge of my plate.

"Don't you live in Los Angeles?" Dad asks.

"I do," I say.

"That's good. You're doing good out there," he says. "Are you going back?"

"I think I'm gonna stick around here for a while," I say.

"Well, whatever you want to do," he says, unrolling the tablecloth and smoothing it beneath his palms. "But don't do it on my account."

I am doing it on Dad's account, but not, I think, in the way he means. I'm here because loving Dad is the thing I do best. At the far end of the little western village in Tinkertown is Boot Hill. The cemetery is filled with tiny tombstones, each painstakingly lettered by Dad. The one for my alter ego Campfire Sally reads, "always there when you needed her." It's a tall order, but I mean to live up to it.

The next morning, I wake up early and take a long, hot shower and get dressed quickly. I pull on black tights even as I know that wearing black tights in New Mexico is a mistake. They act like a magnet for all the dust and dirt and dog hair and pick up as prickly passengers the tiny tri-pointed burrs we call goatheads. I should be wearing leather chaps or at the very least a serviceable pair of jeans, but I feel a need to be pulled together; to cut a slim and authoritative figure, and the only way for me to do this right now is to zip myself into my dark Ann Taylor separates.

Just as I start across the driveway, La comes out the front door of the cottage. She is wearing jodhpurs and tall, brown leather riding boots. Clipped to her belt is the phone from the house. Her hair is wet from the shower.

"Why haven't you opened the gates?" she demands. "We open at nine."

"I gotta say no one's knocking down the door to give us their three dollars."

"But the point is we open at nine."

"I'll get the gate," I say.

"No, I'll get it," she says. She stomps toward the top of the driveway, and I turn and head down toward the museum. Behind me, I hear the hinge on the metal gate screech open.

La's boots crunch down the gravel driveway and hit the boardwalk with a hollow sound as she rushes by me to open the museum door. She clicks open the padlock and pulls the chain through the heart-shaped hole in the blue wooden door of the museum.

I follow La past the bottle walls and down under the porch outside Dad's shop. She stops to push open the door to the Grandma Fortuneteller machine and then continues to the door to the western town. Her head bends in concentration over the padlock as she lines up the numbers.

"Let me do this," I say.

"I don't want to *let* you do it," she says. "I just want you to do it."

I'm still smarting from our fight about dinner last night and so everything she says hits me with a fresh sting.

"You need to get strong, Tanya," she says. "Get it together or get out of here."

"Look," I say, "can you try to be a bit more compassionate? I'm losing my father."

"I don't have time to be compassionate," she says. She yanks the door open and stomps off through the darkened museum.

Back in the house, I splash my face, smooth my hair, and try to collect my things to get to work. There are meetings to go to and brochures to pick up from the printer. The long drive to the North Valley beckons—forty-five minutes alone with my own thoughts and without the sight of La's angry mouth moving in her tight, pointy little face.

From the bathroom, I hear the front door open. I hold my breath and pray for Dad's gentle, measured steps, but hear instead the scurry and hurry of bootfalls that are La's. If I could crawl out the bathroom window right now, I would. Unfortunately, the only way out is through the front door.

"Look," I say, "I have to get to work."

"I just want you to know that I'm disappointed," La responds.

And then I start to shout. I'm not even sure what I'm saying, but I can feel my rage as it surges up out of me.

My mom and dad fought a lot when I was growing up. They fought about how much time Dad spent on the road. They fought about my mother's overzealous volunteer efforts at the zoo. They fought about all the people they each slept with. They fought about almost everything. During one of these fights, my father picked up an antique milk can that we used as a stool in the kitchen and hurled it down the stairs. It hit the wall and took a big chunk out of the plaster. In another fight, my mother started to shake the breakfast table. She knocked over jelly glasses full of orange juice and sent plates skittering onto the lime green linoleum kitchen floor. A different time, my dad stomped out of the house, letting the screen door slam behind him. He collapsed next to me on the front porch. "God, I hate her," he said. I was ten or eleven.

I wonder if it is the ghost of all those fights, the crazy, crackling energy that hovers in the air of this house like smoke after lightning, that makes me want to break a chair over La's head.

"You say you want to help, but what have you done?" La shouts. "There are bulbs out in the museum; there's a bunch of loose boards on the boardwalk. Get a fucking hammer if you want to help."

Living in a museum and running a museum are two different things. I don't know what she wants and she won't take five minutes to tell me.

"Face your danger, Tanya, or get out of here," La yells.

I wrap my fingers around the back of the chair and try to pull myself out of this. I don't want to be fighting. Inside my chest, I can feel my heart like the flapping of a thousand wings.

"Look," I say, "we're all trying to help. It's just that you're running so fast you can't see it."

"I am trying to get everything done," La retorts.

"And so am I. But I need a minute to get my bearings here. I want to help. But it's so hard to see Dad like this."

"I am crazy with sadness, Tan. I don't know what to do except get on with it."

She looks up at me, her blue eyes filled with tears. We face off for a moment and then we kind of lean toward each other. Not quite touching, but somehow at rest.

A couple of days ago I went out to a barn in the North Valley of Albuquerque to hang out with Dad while La took a riding lesson. Her trainer kept telling La to "keep her seat and go the distance." I watched my stepmother level her gaze and grip the reins before digging her heels into Hannah's flank and I felt a sudden burst of kinship with the horse. La seems to need fierce focus to keep her seat and go the distance with Dad. She is running the museum, taking care of Dad, working with a local tourism group to bring more business to Tinkertown and other mountain attractions, and trying to help us get the ad agency off the ground. She is a whirlwind of activity. In her effort to keep moving forward, she's locking down emotionally. I think she expects me to do the same even though I've barely unpacked my suitcase. Although I feel like I'm here to work for her without question, the same way the horse is supposed to jump when she sees a fence, I try to say what I need to say to end this fight.

I have been at the office for only a couple of hours and still feel hoarse from yelling at La when I get a call from Florence. She's in the shop with my dad.

"The old coot's fine," she says. "It's about your Gran."

Grandma Rose had been up visiting for the day when she tripped on the sidewalk in front of the cottage and fell down the three cement steps into the driveway.

"She landed right on her face, the poor thing," Florence says. "Your stepma has taken her to the hospital. I've got to go soon. And I don't think she'd like it if I left old Mister Smarty Pants here all alone with the till."

I can hear my dad's voice in the background and Florence laughs. "He's got a mouth on him still," she says. "I'm sorry to drag you all the way back up here, hon, but I think you ought to come home."

"I'll be there in two minutes."

"It's a forty-five mile drive, miss. We'll see you in an hour."

I make a quick stop at the grocery store and pick up the makings for lasagna. A bagged spinach salad will add some green to our meal tonight and they can all have leftovers for lunch tomorrow. Once I get home, it takes me eight minutes to put the whole thing together. Dad watches as I crack open the jar of sauce and stir the meat in a skillet on the stove.

"Ma took quite a spill," he says. "She's not looking too good."

"How'd it happen?" I ask.

"Oh, you know. She skipped when she should have skapped. She's not quite right up here," he says, tapping his head. "Poor old gal."

La and Grandma arrive home, and I rush out the door to help them out of the car. Grandma looks terrible. She has a huge black and blue bump on her forehead, both eyes are ringed with deep purple bruises, and her nose is cut and crusted with blood. Her glasses were broken in the fall and without them, she looks out at us the way a mouse might look at an owl.

La pours milk for Grandma and Dad and under cover of the open refrigerator door, sloshes wine into coffee cups for the two of us.

"Thanks for making dinner," she says, handing me the cup.

I did not make this tomato sauce from scratch, the noodles are thick and dense, but we are all sitting down together to eat and there is comfort in warm lasagna and in giving over the weight of our bodies to the chairs around the table.

"You're welcome," I say and I touch the rim of her cup with my own.

A Lot of Obstacles * *October 1998*

GRANDMA TELLS ME that there are people eating worms in the basement of Bear Canyon, the "senior community" where she has been living for the past seven months. She does not give this extraordinary news even the emphasis she reserves for the word "different" as in, "that blouse sure is different." Or, "Tattoos, huh? That's different." Bear Canyon does not have a basement.

When we arrange a meeting with the facility manager, a pudgy man in a beige suit, we learn that Grandma has been found wandering the halls, her face blank as a sheet of paper. She has lost her keys. She has missed dinner and seems to have no interest in bingo or a trip to the hair salon. Even before her fall, he says in his honeyed southern accent, he'd begun to question Grandma's ability to "get along in the community."

"Your grandma's a good woman. God knows we just want what's best. But, Lord keep her, Bear Canyon may not be what she needs."

Grandma has broken several bones in her face, but the fall also seems to have broken the last fragile strands connecting her to reality. She spends much of her time sitting in the big wooden rocker, staring out across the yard. She asks me repeatedly when she's going to have to go back to the school.

"You don't have to go to school, Gran," I say. "You can stay here with us."

"Well, I don't mind," she says. "But that horse is getting a little close, don't you think?" She points out into the yard at the barbecue grill.

Dad looks up and says, "Gran's not here so much. There's a lot of obstacles."

It's a funny thing to say, but it's true. She refuses to change out of her pink sweatshirt, and her hair is matted down in the back from sleep and stands out in sticky clumps above her forehead. She looks at us and then pulls herself out of the rocker to look in the wall mirror. She scowls at her reflection as she presses her curls against her forehead, trying to force them flat.

During her months at Bear Canyon, she had a standing appointment at the beauty salon down the hall from her apartment. Once every four or five days, she'd go in for a wash and style, emerging with what Dad called "the George Washington." This sturdy helmet of careful curls was secured with enough hairspray to keep it in place until the next appointment.

"Pee-you," Dad says, holding his nose. "Does she smell or what?"

Gran blinks at him and then turns back to her reflection.

"Dad, stop," I say.

He's right, though, and I'm suddenly sorry we haven't done anything about it before. She's got a doctor's appointment in the morning and even though she doesn't want to change her clothes I think there's still a part of her that would be shocked to go out in public this way.

"Gran, we've got to give you a bath," I say.

She looks forlorn. "A bath?" The word seems utterly foreign.

"Yeah," I say. "I'll run a nice warm bath and you can climb in the tub. It'll be relaxing. Come on, I'll get you started."

I smile and take her arm. I am trying to convince her, but I'm also trying to convince myself. I have no idea how I'm going to get Gran undressed and into the bathtub. The idea of seeing my grandmother naked alarms me.

In the bathroom, I switch on the heat lamp, sit her down on the closed toilet, and kneel to run the water. While the tub fills, I untie her white tennis shoes and slip them off. She's not wearing socks and she wriggles her toes against the rug.

I look up to see Dad leaning against the doorframe. "You're in good hands, there, Ma." He gives me a salute and heads out.

As I begin to pull Gran's sweatshirt over her head, she holds her arms up like a small child. She is not wearing a bra and her breasts are small and pale. Her shoulders fold forward, making her back round and smooth. She stands perfectly still while I take off her slacks. Her cotton briefs are so big the waistband is almost at her sternum. I pull them down, focusing on helping her maintain her balance.

"Are you gonna wash my hair?" she says.

"I am," I say. "And the rest of you too." I take her arm and help her into the tub.

Barely five feet tall, she can extend her legs straight out without touching the end of the tub. I take a washcloth and gently rub it over her back and neck, squeezing out the warm water over her skin.

She looks past me when I hold her arm up to wash her armpit. She is almost completely hairless like a baby. I scrub her back and arms and legs, but I stop when I get to what Gran used to call her "secrets." I have this sudden thought that her vagina, hidden as it is beneath her doughy belly, may have completely disappeared. I'm not ready to find out. I sluice water up between her legs and she does the same.

Gran is wobbly when she stands up and heavier than I think she will be. It's as if she has absorbed the bathwater like driftwood too long in the sea. I take her arm and try to support her weight while she steps out.

I hear the screen door slam followed by the click of La's boots against the brick.

"Well, hello, sweetie," Dad says.

"Where's Tanya?" she says, her voice rising with worry. "Where's Rose?"

She doesn't stop to hear my dad's answer, but instead pulls open the door of the bathroom.

"I gave Gran a bath," I say. "We're okay."

"Well, let's get her dressed," La says. She grabs Gran's clean clothes from the cabinet and starts to pull her shirt over her head. Gran's face pops out the neck hole. Her eyes are wide, her hair is plastered against her forehead.

"I've got it," I say. "It's okay."

"Great," La says. "There's a million people in the museum." And then she's walking again, out of the bathroom and out the back door where her boots crunch quickly across the gravel.

I've begun to realize that part of what makes La move so fast is her belief that she's responsible for everything. She's been running things here for so long that I think she's forgotten how to let anyone help. Leaving me to finish up here with Grandma is a sign of trust. It's progress and I'll take it.

The next day, the doctor tells us that Grandma has Alzheimer's. Though he recommends more tests after her face heals, he is pretty certain she's been experiencing symptoms for years. The move to Albuquerque lifted her like a needle on an old phonograph out of the familiar groove of her life, and so the disease has progressed more rapidly. He is quick to say we shouldn't blame ourselves for her decline.

I think about Grandma's mother, Great-Grandma Blondo. We would visit her in the nursing home when I was a kid. At Grandma's urging, I would sit next to Great-Grandma and let her touch my face with her big, square hands. She would slide her palms over my head, smoothing my hair at the scalp and letting my ponytail slip through her fingers. She spoke only German, and though she lived to be almost one hundred, I never remember a visit where she recognized me, my father, or my grandmother. I think she most likely suffered from Alzheimer's as did Gran's sister, Kate. These are the people I come from. I imagine pushing off their shore in a small boat, looking back as the fog closes in. In front of me is open water with no land in sight.

The doctor suggests that we talk to a social worker, and so I take the morning off work to meet with this tall, careful woman. She wears her blonde hair pulled back from her wide, clear forehead and asks to speak to each of us individually. When it is my turn, she looks right into my eyes.

"You all are in such a difficult place," she says. "You've taken on a lot."

I want to burrow against her and let her stroke my hair. Instead, I blink back tears and sit up straighter. I am facing my danger. "We can handle it," I say. "We're strong."

"Of course you are," she says. "But this is big stuff. Not just your grand-mother, but your father too. It's okay to ask for help."

"Thank you," I say. "Thank you for coming today and for being so calm."

I look across at Grandma. She is nodding in the rocker, her hair standing up on her head like a wire brush above the sunset colors of her face. Just outside, Dad is moving rocks around in the backyard wearing nothing but flip-flops and shorts, his belly hanging over the waistband. La keeps popping in and out of the house. She has both the phone from the cottage and the phone from the Tinkertown house clipped to her belt along with the pager from the gift shop that Maggie and Florence use to let her know when to pick up either line. Her riding boots are dusty and there's a hand-ful of hay in her hair. Car after car pulls down the driveway as more tour-ists line up to hand over their three dollars for a walk through the museum. We are all puffy eyed from crying.

"The show must go on," Dad always said, applying this hardheaded circus philosophy to all situations. The truck broke down? No problem. Fix it. The house burned down? Build a new one. The marriage didn't work? Get out and find a new love. Don't waste energy feeling sorry for yourself. Just get moving.

"Have you thought about a support group?" the social worker asks.

"We have a support group," I say. People accustomed to loss surround us. Florence's daughter Heidi was killed in a car accident, and she loses her husband on a daily basis to alcohol. Maggie's husband died just after they purchased their mountain retirement home. My uncle Louie often drops by with a cooler of beer to sit in the yard with Dad and jaw about the old days when they spent weeks together on the road painting for the carnival. Louie has sad blue eyes and a kind of wistfulness in his voice that makes me feel his greatest loss was the adventure Dad brought into his life. Dad's best buddy Jon Schneck lives in a geodesic dome at the end of a boulder-studded dirt road and welds huge steel sculptures. His back is bent by childhood polio, but he covers his pain with a toothy smile and the loud, rapid-fire laugh of a hyena. My godmother Julie has known Dad since second grade, and sitting at her kitchen table eating tomatoes fresh from her garden feels like support to me. We don't need to find an Alzheimer's group. What we need are people who remember Dad's stories. What we need most are people we can laugh with.

After the social worker leaves, Dad wanders in and stands behind Grandma's rocking chair. He points at her and then taps his head, rolling his eyes. Grandma pulls herself out of the chair and takes a few shuffling steps toward the door.

"Whoa, Ma," Dad says, quickly taking her arm and guiding her gently back to the chair. "You've got to be careful. You're too wobbly."

He settles her carefully in the chair and then backs away, holding his palms facing her. "Stay," he says. "Stay."

She looks out past him and lets out a long, loud fart.

"Eww. Steer clear of Granny Gross Out," he says.

"Dad," I say, "Be nice."

"The fat people need the trust of America and the midgets can eat all they want when it comes from Algeria," Dad says.

"What?" I ask.

"What, what?" he says.

The Alzheimer's books call this jumble of language "word salad," and Dad's been dishing it out more and more regularly. La and I try to write it down the minute he says it because if we wait even a second, it's lost. Our brains are still primed for the logical association of verb and noun. Without that, we have no handle on these sentences, which simply fragment and disappear.

The screen door slams, and Radar and Wallace come racing through, snarling and biting at each other's legs.

"Hey, hey, you monsters," Dad says. "Simmer down." He laughs and follows them as they race out the back door and across the yard. I watch him until he settles into the hammock and folds his hands across his chest. Within seconds, he is asleep.

I turn my attention to tonight's dinner. I am trying to follow La's request for simple things that we can eat for days. I have begun to think of this as "siege food." Tonight we'll have a big pot of white bean chicken chili. Tomorrow we can have it for lunch and probably the next night we'll have it for dinner again. It's not particularly exciting, but it will get us through the next round of shelling.

Grandma Moves Again   * *October 1998*

GRANDMA WILL STAY WITH US until we can move her things out of her apartment at Bear Canyon and into a shared room in a large nursing home called La Paloma Blanca. Jason, Megan, and I volunteer to sort through everything and get rid of all the furniture that was so recently shipped from South Dakota.

Gran's apartment does not seem to be the living space of an addled old woman. There are no dishes in the sink, the bed is made, and the towels are folded neatly on the rack in the bathroom. We don't really know where to start. It's unnerving to be in Gran's home without her.

"What's this crap?" Jason says, pulling a stack of old calendars off the bookshelf. "1984, '88, '92 . . . This is real archival stuff here." As he waves the calendars to emphasize his point, out flutter a handful of five-dollar bills. Jason crouches to retrieve the cash. "Holy shit," he says. "We have to be careful."

We start on the bookcase together. We take out each book, flip through all the pages and then give it a good shake to dislodge anything we may have missed. We find photographs of my dad when he was a baby, carefully folded squares of tissue, bits of fabric, yellowing business cards, giveaway pocket calendars, and cash. Lots of cash. From a Danielle Steele novel, I shake out almost fifty dollars in singles. Folded into the pages of Gran's bible are ten crisp twenty-dollar bills. When we have finished with the bookcase, we have nearly four hundred dollars.

We open scrapbooks and find photos of Grandma in a bathing suit, her knees up, her face tilted coquettishly toward the photographer.

"Do you think she's posing for Grandpa?" Jason asks.

"Probably," I say. But I can't imagine this. My grandfather was gruff and angry, a gray-faced man always wreathed in the stale smells of cigarette smoke and coffee grounds.

"She looks so pretty," Megan says. "So fresh. What happened?"

In a box of scrapbooks, we find a stack of crayon drawings done by Dad when he was four or five. Circus trains and old western towns crowd the pages. The drawings are remarkably detailed and show signs of the artist he will become.

"Christ," Jason says. He holds a drawing of a train leaving a small town in the distance. From the smoke stack are the letters "SOS, SOS, SOS . . ." A cry for help from poor Pop stuck in Aberdeen.

We put all the drawings and scrapbooks in the pile of things to be saved and toss the romance novels in the box for Goodwill.

In a day, we reduce the size of Grandma's closet by two-thirds and sort her possessions into three piles. The trash pile is the largest. The smallest pile is the one filled with things we'd like to keep. There are a couple of patchwork quilts pieced together from squares of heavy wool and polyester in the dark grays and browns of suit fabric. We call them Grandpa pants quilts and joke about their weight. We save Gran's jewelry box and a couple of her old tapestry pocketbooks. There are a few of Dad's early paintings and wood carvings and a little blue sailor suit he wore as a toddler. In the end, everything of value fits neatly in Grandpa's old green army trunk.

Trash bags overflow with pink sponge curlers, wads of tissue, and nylon stockings laddered with runs. We toss twenty-five nail clippers and several bags of hardened candy orange slices. In one of her dresser drawers, we find a ziplock bag filled with the stretchy cuffs of sweatshirts. We are puzzled until we start looking at her sweatshirts and realize that she has shortened almost all of the sleeves, often cutting the cuffs off of one and replacing them with cuffs of a different color.

I am reminded of Christmas ornaments she made out of glitter-encrusted laundry detergent bottle caps and the pencil cases she sewed out of old drapery fabric. Once, when I was nine or ten, I brought her a picture book of fashion throughout history. I circled a bunch of the dresses and asked her to sew them for my dolls. Without patterns, she made ball gowns, fringed flapper dresses, and party frocks with tulip skirts. She was as creative as my father, I realize, even though she never expanded her horizons. I hold the bag of frayed wristbands and think about saving it. I'll stuff it in a box and move it from place to place until one day my kids or grandkids will dig it out, scratch their heads and toss it into the trash. Today, I'll save them the trouble.

The next day, I return to Gran's apartment with my mother. By five o'clock everything has to be out.

"I just want to help," she says. She pokes around in a few of the open boxes and pulls the drawers out in the kitchen.

I drape my arm around her shoulder and give her a squeeze. Only a couple of inches over five feet, she fits against me the way the compact body of a sparrow might fit in my cupped hand. She's wearing a plum-colored blouse and her long, silvery hair runs like mercury down to the middle of her back.

"We packed almost everything yesterday," I say. "Today, there's just the big stuff. If you want anything, you can have it."

"What is there?" she asks. My mother loves to spend Saturdays trolling around Albuquerque, digging through other people's things. She will follow an estate sale sign for miles if she thinks there might be a piece of Stangl pottery or a floral tin tray at the end. Gran's apartment is a kind of garage sale for her, and as much as I believe she really wants to help, a part of me knows that she's in full rummage mode.

"Well, dig around," I say.

I can tell that Mom wants to sit and chat and reminisce about the early years of her marriage with my father, but I don't. Dad's Alzheimer's seems to have rubbed off on Mom as well. It's made her forget all the fights, all the yelling, and all the anger. Now she just wants to relive the good times. But I remember the day she sat in her car and pounded on the steering wheel, screaming in frustration. I see her standing with her back to the fireplace in our living room, her face a mask of sorrow. It was her decision to leave Dad. I think it was a good decision, and it's hard to hear her underplay it.

Mom was angry when Dad married La. Nearly eighteen years later, she's still angry, and a part of me understands why. Both of my parents found comfort in the arms of others, but Dad loved La.

I couldn't side with Mom in the divorce. If I listened to her angry words, I would be betraying my father. If I even let on that I understood her anger, I would be condemning the person I loved best. So I let it go.

In the beginning I loved La because Dad loved La. Later, I loved La because she brought some order into my world. At thirty-two, she had no idea how to parent two kids rocketing toward puberty, and so she turned to books. Consulting titles like *Instant Family*, she set bedtimes, arranged for summer camp, and applied for our social security numbers. She read our report cards and sent away for college information. I had never lacked for love, but I had always craved some organization.

I see now how La with her lithe limbs and blonde hair could be an affront to my sturdy little mom. I can see how her speed might be read as cold and selfish. I vow to be gentler with Mom. I realize she is doing all she can do to help me, and I am grateful.

When I get outside with some of the boxes from Gran's apartment, a few of the residents are starting to take their places on the benches in front of the building.

"Shouldn't a gal like you have a fella to help you out?" a white-haired man in a blue golf shirt asks.

"Should," I say. "But I've got it."

I make a big show of unlatching the tailgate on the truck and muscling the boxes up into the truck bed.

"Yep, looks like you can take care of yourself," he says as I wheel the dolly back inside.

Back upstairs, my mom is in the bathroom holding a bunch of squeezed-out lotions. "I hate to throw these away," she says.

"Then take them home," I say.

"I'll just break out. I'm allergic to almost everything," she says.

"Then toss them," I say.

"You're right," she says. "But doesn't all this make you so sad? I mean, here we are sorting through Rose's whole life and we're just tossing it out like it was nothing."

When my parents divorced, my mom moved out of our house and into a house in Albuquerque. She took a lot of stuff with her in the first move, but every couple of days she would come up while Dad wasn't home and we were at school and take something else. Finally, Dad got sick and tired of her sneaking around and put a padlock on the front door of our house.

"Those things were mine," she said. "We got them when we were together."

When he was on the road, Dad used to work out trades for antiques. Sometimes he'd return after a two-week absence with half a dozen wagon wheels tied to the top of the truck or a couple of beat-up wooden carousel horses leaning against each other under the camper shell. He traded for rewired gas chandeliers, potbellied stoves, turquoise-studded concho belts, a coat made of horsehide, and once a mounted moose head that he hung in our living room. He painted signs in exchange for miner's lamps, dozens of ice tongs, and a pair of dressed fleas. He traded for the iron bed frame where I slept until I went to college and for a pony cart, though we never had a pony.

"More stuff?" my mother would say when he returned home. "But we don't have any money."

Mom still asks about things that were in the house when she was married to Dad.

"Where is my silver concho belt?" she'll ask. "I just can't figure out what happened to it."

I know for a fact that Dad sold the belt to spite her. When he told me, I tried to understand how trapped he felt and I discounted Mom's loss. Now, though, I think that her sentimental attachment was earned as much as Dad's yen for freedom.

I take the bottles from Mom and set them on the counter before slinging my arm around her shoulder.

"We're trying to be sensitive," I say. "We just don't have the space to keep all of this. And she doesn't need it."

"All I hope is that you don't ever have to do this for me," she says.

If I don't, who will? I think. I imagine the number of boxes it will take to hold all the potsherds and tin trays and heart-shaped rocks in Mom's house. I wonder what I will do with her collections of feathers and delicate seashells and bird skulls. Where will I put her bronzed baby shoes and the pink crocheted dress she wore as a child?

We spend the next couple of hours loading the truck with boxes and packing up the last few items. Then I make a dozen phone calls to find the only person willing to pick up Gran's furniture, a soft-spoken man with a pickup truck. He comes alone, and this is how I find myself stuck between the doorframe and the heavy end of Gran's gray Formica vanity.

"I don't think it's going to fit without taking the legs off," he says.

"It'll fit," I say. "It fit when we got it up here." I give it a good shove with my shoulder and we barrel through the door. I think about those women who are able to lift the weight of a truck to free a child or husband. What happens, though, if trucks keep falling on the people you love? Do you always have the strength to pick them up?

That afternoon, I pull the truck around to the back gate of Tinkertown and unload all of Gran's boxes, her rocking chair and her hard-sided blue suitcases onto the back porch. I hope that she is asleep in the cottage and not watching her whole life parade by.

At dinner we explain to Grandma that she'll be moving to a new place called La Paloma Blanca where she'll be sharing a room with a chatty woman called Doris. We've already hung her clothes in the wardrobe and hammered a nail in the wall to hold her crucifix. When her face has healed and her replacement glasses arrive, we'll take her there.

"But what about my things?" she asks. "How will I move all of my things?"

"Well, you know, Ma," Dad says. "You know how in those Christmas movies you see on TV? The ones where you think it's not going to work out, but then an angel takes care of everything? I think it's going to work out a little like that."

Drownproofing * *October 1998*

WHEN I WAKE UP the next morning, sunlight is just starting to break through the windows and Wallace is alert, his eyes staring. I follow his gaze and find nothing. It gives me a shiver because he is clearly seeing something. Wallace cocks his head and whines softly.

I hear a crash from the next room. I jump out of bed, run to the door, and see that the glass ceiling lamp has fallen and broken, littering the floor with milkglass shrapnel.

"Hello?" I say.

"Ghosts and raccoons?" David asks.

"I've got to get rid of the raccoons," I say, shifting the phone to my other ear as I pull a shirt over my head. I'm running late, but I'm still feeling a little shaky and it's easier to be brave when I hear David's voice.

"And a ghost is just fine to float around breaking things?"

"I don't think it's a big deal. It might even be my grandfather looking for Grandma," I say. The big, green steamer trunk parked at the foot of my bed is loaded with odds and ends from their marriage, a distillation of all their years together. "Besides," I add, "there are lots of ghosts in this house. I don't think they're dangerous."

"Okay, now you're freaking me out."

I'm all bluster now as I continue. "I told you about the music, right? The first couple of nights that I was here, I could swear I heard circus music. Like a parade, only really far away."

"Get out of here."

"No, really. La said she's heard the same thing."

"Well, then you're all freaks," David says.

"But you mean that in a nice way, right?" I say.

"Well, sure. But come on. How am I ever supposed to sleep in that house?"

"It's safe," I say.

"That's just what those poor folks at Amityville said."

I tell him that it's not that hard to imagine that my house is haunted. I think of the wedding-cake couple exhibit and the pants and shoes of Louie Moilanen, who at eight feet four inches was once the world's tallest man. Dad's uncle Phil left us hundreds of bullet-shaped promotional pens he collected during his years as a manager for the Piggly Wiggly grocery store. There is a red tuxedo coat with tails that was once worn by the ringmaster in the Sells-Floto circus and a full-length coat made out of dapple-gray horsehair. I imagine all the hands that have touched these objects: the hands of trembling brides as they cut the first slice of cake, the big hands of Louie Moilanen threading the laces through his enormous shoes, the hands of the salesmen who passed those pens to my great uncle Phil, hoping to peddle an extra order of canned vegetables or a few more cartons of cigarettes. If dust is made up primarily of dead skin cells, there is perhaps a finer, lighter dust composed mostly of memory. It is this kind of dust that settles over Tinkertown and filters through the air.

"Look," David says, "I've got a script to put out so I've got to go."

I need to get to work too, but I suddenly feel brushed aside. I realize I've been spinning a yarn, but it's comforting to hear the words spill out. David's abruptness squelches my bravado, leaving me suddenly scared and lonely and flat.

"Right," I say. "Very important business. Bye."

"Wait a second," David says. "You're getting weird on me."

I miss David more than I could have imagined and at the same time, I am angry with him for continuing to have a life without me. This morning, he's already gone to the gym, read the paper, and had his coffee. He doesn't need to tell someone he's okay to feel it.

"Oh, I'm just crazy," I say. "Whatever."

"I don't think you're crazy," David says. "I think you're sad. There's a lot going on, but we can't fix it all right now."

When David was a kid, his dad taught him how to stay afloat in the water without wasting any energy. He learned to kick very gently to the surface for a breath before sinking slightly again. David's dad called this drownproofing and paid David five dollars for every hour that he practiced in the pool. The secret is not to panic, his dad told him.

In our current situation, David seems to be drownproofed. He wakes up early to lift weights and works a long day as a script coordinator at *Buffy the Vampire Slayer*, before heading home to a bachelor dinner of spaghetti with hotdogs or chicken stir-fry. He's writing too: always working on a spec script or a movie idea. And although he spends a fair amount of time wondering if he's a good writer or if we'll stay together, instead of thrashing around in the waves like I do, he takes a calm breath and waits for the future to reveal itself.

"You get going," I say. "I've got raccoons to deal with."

David tells me he loves me. He tells me he believes in me. He tells me that everything is going to be all right. I nod and wipe my eyes and hang up the phone. *In order for it to be all right, I've got to make it all right,* I think. I can't change Dad's diagnosis, I can't be with David. *What can I do?*

I open the phone book to look up the number for animal control. There is little to be done for raccoons, the man on the phone tells me. They're extremely territorial.

"You didn't get this from me," he says, lowering his voice, "but you can try to trap and move them yourself. You could probably get a trap somewhere."

I call around and finally get a line on a guy who says he'll loan me a couple of big live traps if I can come pick them up.

After work, I take the truck and make the journey up over the mountain and down the winding back road into the small town of Placitas. The trap guy lives in a trailer that looks as though it fell out of the sky and into the middle of a field.

"You're sure you know what you're doing?" he asks. "You're just a bit of a girl."

"Shit, yeah," I say, leaning hard on the profanity. I'm driving La's big diesel pickup and instead of my skirt and tights, I pulled on jeans and a pair of black cowboy boots. The boots give me an extra couple of inches and make me walk like I know my way around a ranch.

"Well, if you say so," he says. "Raccoons can be mean. And worse? They're smart. They're like people."

He shows me how to set the big, rectangular trap so that when the raccoon picks up the bait, the door will slam shut behind it. He tells me to click a padlock on the trap after I've caught what he calls "little Houdinis."

When I arrive home, La rushes out, grabs the big cage out of the bed of the truck, and disappears through the gate into the backyard. She's on board for this trapping project. The raccoons have been tearing the shingles off the roof and turning over the flowerpots in search of grubs. They force us to take in the birdfeeders every night or risk broken glass and scattered seed. I know it sounds silly, but it makes me feel connected to her in some deeper way. I am realizing that sometimes the best way to hook into La is to become a fellow adventurer. I climb up into the truck and hand the second trap to Dad.

"What's all this?" he asks.

"Traps," I say. "For the raccoons. They're driving me crazy."

"Poor fellas," he says. "They're just getting their house in order and here you women come with your big boots and your big traps . . ."

"It's not their house," I say.

"It's my house," Dad says. "At least it used to be."

It's nearly ten and I'm in the purple kitchen slicing up apples and opening a can of dog food. It doesn't look that appealing so I add a handful of cereal and a couple of spoons of peanut butter and stir the whole thing together. I head outside to the back porch and smear the mess onto the trap's bait plate.

I try to sleep, but I am too nervous. I try to read, but I can feel my body coiled in anticipation. Usually, when I can't sleep, I close my eyes and wait for my brain to give me a number. I'll let myself go blank for a second and then a number will come: 87, 165, sometimes as low as 41 or 36. If I count backward from this number, I am always asleep before I reach the number one. Tonight, I close my eyes and wait for my number to float out of the darkness, but all I see is the face of Dr. Gorman, Dad's neurologist. When we met with him just after Dad's diagnosis, he unscrewed a ballpoint pen and showed us the spring inside. The drug Aricept, he said, would hold Dad's memory—for a while, at least—like a spring under pressure. But once it stopped working, as it inevitably would, his memory loss would accelerate. He opened his fingers and the spring popped out and rolled off his desk onto the floor.

I don't have any tools to deal with this kind of loss. David has his drownproofing, but I grew up in a landlocked state and I have never been a good swimmer. No one has explained how to float to safety and so I am taking charge here in the only way that I can. When La was my age, she built her own house on a ranch up in Northern New Mexico. She lived alone for two winters. She knows how to fix a pipe, how to wire a lamp, how to tar a roof. She can chop wood and build fires and make a pot of chicken soup that will last for a week. I know how to prepare a soufflé and knit a scarf, but I don't think that is the stuff that's going to get me through this experience. She may not have time for compassion, but La is getting the job done. I need to prove that I can too.

It's after one in the morning when I finally hear the trap slam shut. I pull a sweatshirt over my flannel pajamas and rush out onto the porch with a lock in hand. I play my flashlight over the trap and catch a glimpse of the animal inside. I've caught a big male. He's so big he stoops in the cage and bares his teeth when the light hits his face. My heart is beating as I grab a padlock and approach the cage. He hurls his body against the bars as I take a deep breath and hold the lock out. As soon as it touches the edge, the raccoon grabs it out of my hands and throws it into the back of the trap. I am so startled I drop the flashlight.

"Fuck," I say. "This isn't your house."

I see a piece of nylon rope by the back door and I grab it, thinking maybe I can tie the cage shut. The raccoon growls as I reach out with the rope and runs around in a circle, banging its body against the sides of the trap as I thread the rope through the door and a section of the wall. As I pull both ends tight and begin to tie a knot, the raccoon grabs the rope and pulls back hard. I hold on and we are in a tug of war, him snarling and me swearing. The wind is blowing and the flashlight is rolling over and over, finally catching the eyes of three more raccoons as they come up over the edge of the porch.

"No fucking way," I say.

I am distracted for a second by the approach of the cavalry, and the raccoon inside takes full advantage and pulls the rope through the bars and inside the cage. He has my lock, he has my rope. He has allies. I grab my flashlight and run inside. In the time it takes me to slide the lock on the back door into place, the raccoon has escaped. I watch his silvery body disappear into the night before scurrying back to my bed. If they can get out of the cage, I think, what's to stop them from getting in the house? When I finally collapse into sleep, my dreams are full of skittering shapes and grasping damp fingers.

The next morning, I wake to La's footsteps on the back porch. I jump out of bed, throw on a sweater, and head out to meet her. I am disappointed that I can't present her with a raccoon, but I do have a pretty good story.

"Hey there, good morning." She is wearing one of Dad's denim shirts over her nightgown. Goosebumps dot her thin legs. "I heard the dogs," she says. "Did you get one?"

"I did, but he managed to escape."

I tell La about my midnight tug of war and show her how the raccoon threw the lock back into the cage.

"They've got serious backup," I say.

La puts her arm around me. "Bet you didn't expect this, huh?"

I'm not sure what exactly she's talking about, but I lean into her a little. She's not much for hugging. Sometimes she'll kind of grip my arm or my shoulder and give me a squeeze. It's rough affection, the kind you'd give a horse or a big dog.

"I'm up to it," I say.

La gives my shoulder one final rub with her thumb and starts toward the gate.

"I know," she says. "I have faith."

We Settle into a Routine * *November 1998*

THE MUSEUM IS CLOSED for the season. Without the daily need to open the gate, La seems to have calmed down. She's moved the horse to a barn in Albuquerque for the winter and structures her days around riding lessons. Though Dad seems to miss the visitors, he is just as happy to spend his days trailing after La or sitting in the bleachers at the horse ring, his head bent over a sketchbook. He fills page after page with drawings of Radar and Wallace and La and Gene Autry. He writes in rhyme and refers to himself as "the geezer," or the "old geek." He makes lists. He reminds himself to "Laff if U Can."

At night, the arrival of the new television season has helped us to get into a routine. On Mondays, it's *Ally McBeal*. After dinner, I put the kettle on, and La settles into the couch with her legs stretched out across Dad's lap. I usually share the butterscotch-colored armchair with Wallace or Nick, the huge, old, one-eyed tabby.

"What's the deal with *Ally McBeal*?" Dad asks again and again, savoring the rhyme.

On Sundays, we gather for *Masterpiece Theater* or *Mystery!*, and on many other nights, we rent movies. Dad develops an intense hatred for Christopher Walken.

"That asshole," he says. "I can't even watch that guy. He's some sort of murkamurk. He's fiddling and piddling and evil weevil. Fuck that guy."

Later he develops the same animosity for Phillip Seymour Hoffman. When we go to the movie theater to see *The Talented Mr. Ripley*, he applauds when Hoffman's character is bludgeoned to death.

"The best part of the whole deal was getting rid of that asshole," he says afterward.

The one film we count on to keep Dad cheerful and amused is *The Greatest Show on Earth*. Dad's seen the film many times and has memorized huge chunks of dialog. He recites the lines just a few beats ahead of the actors, often giving me a wink as if to say, "the old man has still got it." He tells me that the circus band will never play "Stars and Stripes Forever," unless it's an emergency. He tells me the ringmaster's horse is named Starless Night. He imagines how much the real circus people must have hated having all the actors in their tent. He can tell, he says, that the real clowns don't want anything to do with Jimmy Stewart.

"Look at that poor guy," Dad says as Stewart tries to ham it up with the legendary clown, Emmett Kelly. "He just doesn't know who he's supposed to be."

It's strange to be spending all our time gathered around the television. We rarely watched television when I was growing up. Instead, we'd join Dad in the shop for what he called Tinkertown Nights, where he'd work on his most current project and Jason and I would take sandpaper to a team of wooden horses or a few more carved figures. Other nights, we'd sit together, each lost in our own book. I read *The Black Stallion* and *A Wrinkle in Time* while Dad meandered through the 1930s and '40s in his collection of *Desert Highways* magazine. Even then, his sense of time seemed more fluid than ours. More than once, he'd put down the magazine and place a call to someone mentioned in a decades old article. Sometimes, he'd find only a disconnected number, but more often, he'd spend an hour or so talking to the owner of a mining museum or a self-described "rock-hound recluse."

"Well, what do you know?" he'd say, hanging up the phone. "The old place is still in business."

For Dad, television, like his magazines, was a window to the past. He often let me stay up past my bedtime so that I could see *Singin' in the Rain*, *Top Hat*, or Betty Grable in *Coney Island*. Dad had seen most of these movies for the first time on the big screen at the Orpheum Theatre in Aberdeen.

"Fifteen cents for a movie ticket and a dime for a bag of popcorn," he'd say. "What a deal."

He talks more and more about those days in Aberdeen. He tells stories about his friend Gary Anderson, a boy with polio who moved away when Dad was in second grade.

"God, I miss that guy," Dad will say, wiping his eyes. "He was a real friend." That this childhood loss could feel so fresh is unnerving. I can feel the past moving forward in Dad's mind, devouring his present. In a life spanning nearly sixty years, I am recent. I feel a strange kind of anger at all those schoolyard friends and army buddies from Dad's youth. Will he remember them when he's forgotten me?

"What are you looking at?" Dad snarls at me when I catch him drinking a beer back behind the old Jeep Cherokee-turned-"art car."

"Is that warm?" I ask, trying to be light.

"It's just fine," Dad says, swallowing the rest and tossing the bottle over-hand into the trees. "And now it's gone. Are you gonna report back to her?"

"Her who?" I ask.

"Oh, you know," Dad says.

"I just don't think you should be drinking," I say.

"Well, try just not thinking," Dad says. He pulls the keys out of his pocket and jumps into the driver's seat of the Jeep.

"You shouldn't drive," I say. "Where do you want to go? I'll take you."

Dad turns the key and guns the engine.

"You can't get there," he says, and then he steps on the gas and blazes out of the driveway, leaving me in a cloud of dust.

La runs out of the house and joins me in the driveway.

"I'm sorry," I say.

"It's not your fault," she says. "I keep thinking I should disable the car, but I hate to do it. It's like clipping his wings."

La and I call a few friends around the mountain and ask them to keep an eye out for Dad. And then we wait. About an hour later, we hear the Jeep before we see it. The engine is roaring and when Dad turns into the drive-way, there's smoke billowing out from beneath the hood.

La and I run into the driveway and find Dad wide-eyed and confused.

"It's gone wacky," he says. "Something turned and snapped and it's fucked."

"You can say that again," La says, popping the hood and peering through the smoke. "Looks like the fan belt broke."

Dad wipes his eyes with the back of his hand, his shoulders sagging. La slams the hood and takes Dad's hand, guiding him into the cottage. He's mild and calm now, the angry wind all blown out.

Later, when Dad has fallen asleep, La and I roll the Jeep back into its parking spot under the shed and lift the hood. We disconnect the wires from the alternator and turn Dad's wheels into a permanent exhibit in the museum. We don't say much. Without wheels, Dad is one step closer to death and we know it.

One night we are curled in front of the television in the cottage and Dad looks up at La and me as though we are strangers.

"I'm like a man with two brains," he says. "There's the part that is with me and the part that travels and changes. I know what I'm doing and then I don't and it goes and it goes and it goes like that."

He is laughing, but he seems scared too. I want to reach for my pen to commit this particular ramble to paper, but I am afraid to move. For one fragile moment, he is completely aware of what is happening to him. I can see how frightening it is. He is no longer in control. He is not paging through magazines, or turning the channel to find an old movie, his brain is flipping through memories like a slide projector gone haywire. He's lost the keys to the car and from here on something else has taken the wheel.

The Bird House * *January 1999*

GRANDMA ROSE HAS BEGUN to hit people. She has also begun to swear.

Gran has been living at La Paloma Blanca for a little over six months. The name means "the white dove" and is supposed to conjure up images of peace and calm. Dad always calls it the bird house, which brings to mind the constant rustle of feathers, the scrape of beak and claw. The place is big and white with a series of long, linoleum-covered hallways radiating out from a central nurse's hub. Grandma shares her room with a chatty woman named Doris, who is confined to a wheelchair and delights in windy descriptions of her grandchildren.

Grandma's closet is filled with the bright blues and pinks and reds of her exclusively polyester wardrobe. She has a television and a reading lamp and a framed drawing of her namesake flower, the rose. We pin photos of distant relations on her bulletin board and read their letters aloud. We say, "You remember Margie, don't you?" When we visit, we say, "SO-AND-SO says hello."

I cannot imagine my own feet in worn slippers shuffling down this shiny linoleum hallway. I cannot imagine that sleep would come easily to a narrow bed set on wheels. Any person fit enough to drive up to the place is going to feel the uncomfortable grip of mortality clamp down the second they step through the door. I rarely meet another visitor, and I understand why. I have to summon the will to step back and see that Gran is safe here. But it is hard not to notice the scent of urine, lurking just under the sharper, piney scent of disinfectant. I think about the aides pushing hampers filled with soiled sheets through the hall. I wonder what it is like to fall asleep and wake up in a place filled with strangers. I begin to think that confronted with the same situation, I might begin to hit people too.

Though she has forgotten that I am her granddaughter, I am still a familiar presence and so when I visit, Gran greets me with a smile. One day I find her sleeping in a chair near the nurse's station. I kneel next to her and tap her gently on the shoulder. She shifts and then sits up straight. I adjust her glasses and take her hands in my own.

"Hi," I say.

"Hi, yourself," she returns.

She stands, all business, and walks to a large, red metal file cabinet.

"You hungry?" she asks.

"Not really."

"Well, let's see what we've got in the icebox."

She pulls on the drawers of the cabinet, but they don't budge. The cabinet is locked.

"Something's wrong," she says. "It's broke or something."

"You know," I say, "I meant to call the guy about that. What do you say we take a walk and see if we can find something to eat?"

"Sure," she says. "Maybe that place across town."

"Which place?"

"You know the one."

"I do," I say and take her arm so that we can walk down the hall together. As we walk, she nods at the nurses and other residents. We pass a man in a wheelchair, and Gran slows for a minute. Her face softens and her eyes grow bright. She takes my elbow and leans in conspiratorially.

"He was there again last night when I got home, sitting out on the lawn."

"Who?" I ask.

"Him. Even though I told him when I left that I'd be mad as hell if I ever saw him again."

She's trying to hide a smile. Gran is clearly pleased. I wonder if she's remembering my grandfather.

"Was it Everett?" I ask.

She ignores my question and walks on. I let it drop. Alzheimer's disease is like a slot machine. You pull the handle and, with a little luck, sometimes things line up. When they do, it's hard for me not to play along. In today's jackpot, file cabinets are refrigerators, the halls have become streets, and Gran is nineteen again playing at being a heartbreaker in her old hometown.

I like these visits with Gran. I feel closer to her now. She has always kept things tight and small, meting out kisses and information with the same miserly control. Now, though, Alzheimer's has loosened her, and she is springing to life. She tells me secrets, talking to me like I'm one of the "girls." I think of the black-and-white photos of Grandma posed coyly in a swimsuit that we found when we emptied her apartment. Her eyes held the same spark that I have always seen in Dad's. Though Alzheimer's disease can be violent as a tornado, wiping out everything in its path, with Grandma, right now, it seems to be blowing softly, coaxing to life a spark long gone cold.

On another visit, I bring Dad. The three of us sit in the common room and watch a cage of finches chatter and hop from branch to branch.

"What do you think of those birds?" I ask, but today Grandma is silent. She takes the fabric of my coat sleeve between her fingers and examines it.

"That's a real nice fabric. What kind of fabric is that?"

"It's velvet," I say.

Dad sighs heavily, slides his sleeve up, looks at his bare wrist and says, "We should hit it."

"In a minute," I say.

"It's getting late," he says. He leans over and pats Grandma on the knee. "We've got to get going now, Ma."

She looks up at him. "Why didn't little Ross come?" she asks.

"All right, enough's enough," he says. "Let's get the hell out of here."

I kiss Grandma on the head and follow Dad across the room, down the hall, and into the clear air outside. When we reach the car, Dad stops and stares at me hard. "Can you believe that? Little Ross? I'm Ross. She doesn't get it. I'm never coming back to this hellhole."

"You don't have to if you don't want to," I say. He is angry today because his mother didn't remember him. I can't imagine how I'll feel when he doesn't remember me.

"Is this our car?" Dad asks.

"Sure is," I say. I unlock his door and help him in, reaching across to fasten his seatbelt. Things like latches and seat-belt fasteners have begun to baffle him, so it's easier if I do it quickly before he gets frustrated. I'm wondering if it was a good idea to bring him here today. Though we all try to talk around it, Grandma's stint in La Paloma Blanca is a kind of dress rehearsal for what we will encounter with Dad. When I think about this for too long, I get a tight feeling in my chest. I unlock my own door and climb in beside Dad. He's rummaged around in the glove compartment and found a pen and a few napkins. Using his knee as a table, he hunches over the napkin, sketching out a scene. With a few strokes of his pen, the desert sky stretches vast and endless over a narrow highway, curving briefly over the sand before becoming lost in the horizon. Is that empty road the one we're on?

The Tattoo Project * *February 1999*

"HEY, HERE'S A LITTLE SOMETHING for the tattoo kid," Dad says. He leans a pen and ink drawing against my oatmeal bowl. "You gonna see your wild brother today?"

"I don't know," I say. "I never know where he's going to be."

"Well, if you see him, give him this, will you. Tell him I want to set up some time to get back under the needle."

Up until a few months ago, despite all his years on the carnival, Dad only had one tattoo, a small green lizard on his chest done by a man known only as Singapore John. Now, though, he's got three new pieces all done by my brother and ideas for a dozen more. First was a brightly colored poster for the Sells Floto circus on his shoulder. His skin had barely healed before he was back in the studio asking Jason to add the logo from The House on the Rock, a roadside attraction in Wisconsin and one of Dad's favorite places on the planet. He added a black-and-white portrait of his mentor, Don Poblo, a drawing of Radar, and a naked woman reaching for a sun just between his shoulder blades.

"That's my sweetie," he said.

La shrugged. "I don't think it looks like me at all."

More tattoos followed in quick succession, including a group of nudists jumping off a dock that he cut off the masthead of the *Skinny Dipper* newsletter.

Dad is relying on his body to remember what his brain cannot. He started with the big things like the circus, the Old West, and his family, but now he's progressing to silly, strange things that catch his ever-wandering attention. When he added the skinny dippers, La wondered if he was really thinking things out. She wondered whether he ought to take a break. So did I.

I think about what I would want tattooed on me. If I were to entrust my memory to my skin, I might start with a tattoo of Dad. Maybe an illustration of a book to celebrate my love of reading. What would represent my talent for writing? A pen or typewriter or my unromantic laptop. Eventually, I might get down to the angel-food cake I like for my birthday, the elbow noodles in a good batch of macaroni and cheese, or the outline of my favorite pillow. The list could grow and grow until everything that influenced me would be written across my body like the ingredients on a box of cereal.

My brother learned to tattoo when he was in college. While he learned, he started his own collection. Beginning with a black tribal band around his arm, his illustrated body now includes an Aztec butterfly symbol broad as two hands emblazoned in red and black on his stomach, a portrait of Frida Kahlo on his calf and, as a Mother's Day gift to our own mother, "Mom" inscribed on a ruby heart. He began piercing parts of himself as well, opening up holes in his earlobes until they grew from the diameter of a chopstick to the size of a quarter.

On one of Jason's early visits to Los Angeles, he told me the one thing he really wanted to do was go to a piercing studio called The Gauntlet and get a Prince Albert.

"I want them to pierce my action," he said. He peered at me to make sure I understood.

"Oh, sure," I said, trying to be nonchalant.

"You know, my penis," he said, when he could tell that I didn't.

"You're sure you don't want to go to Disneyland?" I asked.

Still trying to be cool, I accompanied him to the studio and sat on a sundeck with a cigarette while the piercer ran a razor sharp, hollow needle through some part of my brother's "action." The receptionist, a bald woman with at least twenty silver rings piercing various parts of her scalp, joined me outside.

"I watched," she said. "It's a rare piercing. What a treat for you, though."

"What do you mean?" I asked.

She lifted one studded brow and leaned toward me, so close I could see the smudge of lipstick on her front incisor. "It's very satisfying sexually," she said.

"He's my brother." I was quick to correct her, but I was oddly flattered that she would think a girl like me would have such a cool boyfriend.

"So tell Jason he's got a date," Dad says. He taps the drawing of a mining town. "He's gonna love this one."

Dad may be trying to hold on to the things that mattered to him, but I think this tattoo project is also about Jason.

Jason inherited my dad's magic hand and his way with women. He grew to be as tall as Dad and shares his fondness for beer and a good story. He has an easy way of talking to anyone while at the same time keeping his own counsel. Jason is fidgety without a project, his hands always reaching for a pencil, a carving knife, or a tree saw. As a tattoo artist, he is as close to "with it" as he can be without letting the road take him away from Megan. I wonder if it is their similarity that has always kept my dad and my brother apart.

Jason picks up Dad on his motorcycle and rides him off to the tattoo studio where they sit and bullshit with the rest of the guys in the shop and let the afternoon roll on by.

I can see that Dad is trying to make up for lost time. I have no doubt that he has always loved my brother as much as he loves me, but I know it was not always easy for him to show it. Now he's found a way for them to be together, and he is reveling in this new relationship. I am grateful that they are trying to mend fences. Over the years I have spent so much energy trying to defend Dad to Jason, trying to explain away his slights and point out his good heart, that I am glad Jason will get a chance to see it for himself.

Of course, I can't help but be a little jealous. Jason's not the one shaking out medicine into his palm for Dad to swallow in the morning; he isn't here for the lashing when a few secret beers sharpen Dad's tongue. From Dad's point of view, "care" is looking a lot like "limits," and so I am relegated to playing Nurse Ratched while Jason takes over as best kid.

The Escape Artists * *March 1999*

DAD HAS GROWN SLIPPERY as an eel lately, disappearing so quickly we don't realize he's gone. Though we've caught him twice on the road half-way between the house and the new gas station, once he managed to make it all the way there, returning with a bag of barbecue potato chips and a six-pack. Before we knew what happened, he'd pounded down three beers. Red-cheeked and belligerent, he yelled at La and me when we asked him where he'd been.

"Fuck this," he said, turning away from us and stumbling out into the yard.

We left him alone and a few minutes later saw that he'd fallen asleep in a chair in the backyard with Radar curled tight at his feet.

I can see why he'd be angry with us. We're constantly telling him to stay put, eat his dinner, take his medicine. When he returns to the house after fruitless attempts to start the engine of the Jeep, we let him call our friend Maury the mechanic. Maury is in on our deception and always claims to be real busy. "Next week at the earliest," is all he can promise. Because Dad is forgetting so much, he never stops to question why next week never comes. So, instead of driving, he just takes off on foot attempting another gas station beer run.

Grandma, too, has become something of an escape artist. Though she's been fitted with a bracelet that renders the front doors of La Paloma Blanca inoperative when she approaches, she still manages to make her way out into the parking lot a couple of times a week. She's grown sly, as though her brain, divested of memories, has homed in only on the need for freedom. She hovers near the front door, staring off into the distance until a visitor punches in the code from the outside. As soon as the door is open, she springs to life and heads out like a busy homemaker with errands to run. Once she reaches the parking lot, her momentum slows. She is often found wandering in a small circle or sitting on a bench with her head in her hands. Freedom achieved is nothing without the ability to plot the next move.

With only the music of Hank Williams to keep him company and the red and blue lines in the road atlas for a guide, Dad traveled what he liked to call "the highways and byways" of the whole United States. Grandma, in her tightly tied headscarf and sensible shoes traveled only a mile or two on her daily walks through Aberdeen, but they both, at one time, were able to steer themselves safely through the world. Now we contemplate what's called a locked unit for Grandma, and, although we don't speak of it, we know one day Dad may need a place like this too.

Megan and I take the day off from the ad agency to look at Alzheimer's care facilities in Albuquerque. We stop first for coffee and then run into the fancy tobacconist for imported cigarettes. Slim and wrapped in candy-colored paper, they are strong enough to make me a little lightheaded. In the car, Megan selects a bright pink one, lights up and rolls down the window. Strands of her reddish hair glisten as they escape from her barrette.

"Poor guy," she says, pointing ahead to a dead prairie dog. I swerve and as I do, I run over a second one. The tires bump-bump over his soft body.

"Holy shit," I say.

"He was probably going to check on the other one," she says. "It's for the best. Now they're together."

It's macabre, but we start to laugh. As we continue down the road, I can't help but feel a little like that prairie dog, running across the road, dodging cars to check on my fallen family members.

At the first couple of homes we visit, we hop out of the car bright with hope. But after finding dimly lit hallways, grimy linoleum, and the blank stares of old men in hospital gowns, we quickly become discouraged. I had hoped the term "locked unit" would belie the cozy haven inside, but each of these places seems more Cuckoo's Nest than the one before.

In comparison to the other places, Manor Care seems like a resort. It is small, just two hallways connected in a V at the nurse's center. There is a nice patio and a common room with cheerful pink furniture and a big kitchen that smells of freshly baked cookies.

We rattle through our family saga and try to ignore the director's widening eyes when we explain about both Gran and Dad. I don't know why she's so surprised. All the Alzheimer's books tell you to "expect the unexpected," and we are exactly that. We run through payment options and visiting hours and peek in one of the wardrobe cabinets assigned to the patients. (The director assures us she'd rather call them clients.) We will not have to do much packing for Gran in this last transition. In the same way it steals words and logic, the disease has robbed her of possessions if only by removing her ideas of ownership and attachment. When I think of it like this, it is harder to imagine Dad living here. He is so solidly attached to Tinkertown. In the museum, his thoughts and memories are on display for everyone to see. With a kind of prescient instinct, he built a walk-through scrapbook that, at least as I imagine it, is helping him stay with us as long as he can.

Back home that night, La makes a fire in the cottage woodstove and we sit together after dinner. Dad is on the far end of the sofa, his head bent over his sketchbook. La snuggles next to him, tucking her feet up under her robe. She is pleased that I helped find a place for Gran and I am happy to have taken something off her plate. Wallace sleeps on his back in the dog bed next to the stove, offering his belly up to the warmth, and Radar circles and circles at Dad's feet before tucking his nose tightly against his tail and closing his eyes.

Outside, the sky is ink black and the shape of the mountain just a shade darker. In the forest, decades of shed pine needles form a mulchy surface that gives slightly under a boot. Scratch it aside and you find red earth and below that, hard bedrock that bears the imprint of shells and sea creatures. In the company of my parents, I learned to search for these fossils. In the Tinkertown house is the dress I wore to my sixth birthday party and the letter accepting me to college. The quilts Grandma made are there too, folded in a trunk along with her photo albums and jewelry. Everywhere around me are signs of the past, but I can only guess at what is coming next.

On the sofa, La has nodded off. Dad lifts his eyes from his sketchbook, gently removes her reading glasses, and then continues to draw. There is no need for locks now, we are held here inside the house by the warmth and comfort of each other.

Dad's Birthday * *April 1999*

DAVID TAKES A YARDSTICK and makes a grid on a large piece of newsprint. One of Dad's drawings of Radar is propped against a wineglass on the table in front of him.

"You want it to look right or not?" he asks, catching a glimpse of my smirk.

"Of course. It's just that you're being so careful."

"I think we all know," David says, "that I'm not one of you weird mountain freehand freaks."

I smile and take a sip of wine. The air is sweet with chocolate. When the cake cools, David will cut it into the shape of Radar and frost it white for Dad's birthday. Though this was my idea, David jumped on board immediately. He is a cake guy. He brought a rum Bundt on our first official date and copied a watermelon-shaped ice cream bombe from the pages of Martha Stewart for my thirtieth birthday.

I watch as he carefully transfers Dad's drawing to the large grid, filling in the big ears and wide, cartoon eyes of "the best dog in the world." Tonight's party was La's idea. A "blowout," she called it. "Just a big, fun event while your dad can still enjoy it. I don't think we'll have many more parties here."

We hear the rattle of the front door latch and look up from the table to see Dad. He gives us a wave and wanders into the kitchen and opens the fridge. He's eating a lot lately. I don't think he's any hungrier than usual, he just forgets. At lunch a couple of days ago, he ate a huge chicken burrito and methodically mopped all the chile sauce from the plate with an extra tortilla. A few seconds after he'd popped the last morsel into his mouth, he looked down at his plate and said, "So, what's for lunch?"

I set our wine glasses down on one of the chairs where they are hidden by the tablecloth. "Do you need something?" I ask.

"Need? Need?" he says. "Oh, I don't know."

He closes the refrigerator and comes to stand in the opening between the kitchen and the big room that holds both the couch and the dining room table. He squints at David's drawing and then comes down the steps to pick up his own drawing of Radar.

"Now this is a good one," he says.

"We're making a cake," I say, since I don't have to worry about ruining the surprise.

The party is in full swing. I'm wearing a short black dress and my bare arms feel cool and free. Spring is coming, and it's nice to get out from under the wooly layers of winter. It seems everyone has hauled out the mountain finery. My friend Nilz sports a thrift-store western-style suit that smells a bit musty, as though it had been recently lifted from Roy Rogers's trunk. Jason's iridescent sharkskin shirt shimmers in the light. There are bolo ties and turquoise earrings to spare, and wherever I point my camera, I am met by a toothy grin. Though we set out with a kind of grim determination to make this party a good one, I have the happy realization that there is no way to get all of these people in one room without having a good time.

David meets me in the kitchen with a box of birthday candles and as we quickly poke a few through the white frosting on the Radar cake, I am reminded of all the crazy cakes my parents used to create for Jason and me. There were huge sugary castles and dinosaurs and, once, a log-ride cake with real wooden logs going down a bright blue frosted waterfall. I doubt that David will ever build a bottle wall or paint our refrigerator purple. It is unlikely that he will trade a day's work for a covered wagon and even more unlikely that he'll tattoo his body with a collection of his favorite things. But I know for a fact that he would be willing to construct miraculous cakes for our children.

For a long time, I was looking for a boyfriend who was as passionate about things as my dad. I got involved with men who collected pinball machines or who ignored my phone calls to spend the day working on their novel. I was once given a potbellied pig when what I really wanted was a dog. I thought somehow that I needed the eccentricity and unpredictability of my father to make me happy. But I think what I really was looking for was someone to love me as completely as my father does. David is that guy. He hands me the cake and with his voice in my ear, I turn toward the living room. Everyone begins to sing the birthday song and Dad stands up and claps his hands together like a child.

"Oh, boy," he says.

I set the cake on the table in front of him and he wraps his arm around me and gives me a tight hug. As the song ends, everyone applauds and whistles.

"This is a great time," he whispers in my ear.

My eyes fill up and I hug him back hard.

Bob Dylan plays on the stereo while Dad opens presents. La stays close, leaning in to peel a bit of tape, help with a knot of ribbon, or read the first few lines of a card. She holds a white, plastic trash bag, moving quickly to clear away wrapping paper. The gifts are mostly toys. A parade of wind-up cars and rubber chickens. There is a small plastic dog and a bag of candied orange slices and a button bearing the face of Alexander Calder.

"More, more," Dad says after each gift is unwrapped. "This kind of garbage is what keeps Tinkertown growing."

Dad holds the next box for a moment too long. His eyes, which were bright with laughter, have gone blank and bland. He's forgotten what he's doing. La swoops in and peels back the paper. Dad looks up at her for a beat and then clicks back in. The light returns to his face and he slides his glasses down on his nose and looks out at the crowd.

"You know," he says, "Carla takes care of me now that I'm all full of Alzheimer's. Hell, she even comes in and picks my nose for me."

La's teeth clench nervously as she takes a quick breath. He's had a couple of beers and I know she is wondering what he'll say next. Is this where the evening is going to take a turn for the worse?

"I'd like to set my head on fire . . ." Dad says.

La suddenly leans down and interrupts him with a big kiss. When she pulls away, the gleam has returned to Dad's eyes.

"Everyone's been so wonderful," Dad says. "How come life is so weird?"

For the grand finale, Dad unwraps himself. He suddenly stands and takes his shirt off to give our guests a tour of his tattoos. He explains that the logo for the "Skinny Dippers" nudist society can also be found on coffee cups. The needle has lifted off the Dylan album and the room gets very quiet as Dad explains that Jason did "a hell of a job" on the tattoos. In a serious tone, as though he is outlining a city expansion plan, he tells us that there will be a herd of horses running from his shoulder across his chest and trailing down around his legs. "I'm not kidding," he says. "If you really want to go nuts, go crazy."

I look around the room and see that Megan's eyes are red. She leans against Jason, who runs his fingers through her short hair. As hard as we've tried to keep it out, Dad's illness is forcing its way back in and draining the life from the party.

"One of these days when you pass away," Florence says suddenly, "Carla's gonna have your hide tanned. It's the history of Tinkertown."

"You know what? I'm not going anywhere," Dad says.

Later, after everyone has gone home, David wanders around the house picking up empty glasses while I watch the video from the party on the tiny screen of my camera. The house appears darker than it is in life, and bigger. The sound goes in and out, the laughter in the room often louder than anything else. Suddenly, I'm on the screen, the dark line of my bobbed hair a sharp contrast against the pale skin of my neck. When I turn to find myself caught in the lens, I smile. My smile is so wide, so unabashedly filled with joy, that I rewind and watch it again.

"Watch this," I say to David.

"You're gorgeous," he says, peering at the tiny screen.

"Look at how I look at you," I say.

"I look at it all the time," he says. "I like it."

Out with the Folks * *May 1999*

DAD WANTS TO GET BACK ON THE ROAD. He wants to travel to every major amusement park in the country to ride the giant wooden roller coasters. He wants to make it back to Texas to see the Cadillac Ranch. He'd like to get back up to Wisconsin for a tour of The House on the Rock. We sit in front of La's computer and search "art cars" and "carnival" and "folk art."

"What I'd like to see are some nudist camps," Dad says.

"Um . . . really?"

"Yeah, can you type 'nudist colony' into that new-fangled machinery there, Daughter?"

"Sure," I say. It's hard for me to deny Dad anything these days. Why bother to say no when he's got so little time and still so much enthusiasm?

As soon as I hit "enter," though, I realize my mistake. At first, we come up with a few sites showing earnest folks with pale skin and long hair.

"Hit that one," Dad says, reaching for the mouse. He clicks a button and we're confronted with an image of two "schoolgirls" engaged in a bit of extracurricular activity.

"Will you look at that?" Dad reads the screen. "Hot, hot, hot."

"Yep, and I think we're going to have to shut 'er down," I say, punching the off button and sitting back in my chair.

Dad wants to travel to the circus museum in Baraboo and take a trip out to San Francisco to eat an omelet at the Cliff House and throw a few quarters into the ancient fortune-telling machines in the arcade downstairs.

"Hell, I'd just like to get out of Dodge for a while," he says. "Watch the sky, pedal to the metal, and fuck the world."

"Sure," I say. "Let's go."

"Well," he starts, "she'd miss us. And old Radar here, he'd sure miss us. I guess maybe another time . . ."

Though we travel all over the world and see all kinds of things on the Internet, our actual road trips only take us into Albuquerque, where we walk the aisles of a big craft store called Hobby Lobby. We spend ages checking out paint and fake flowers and scrapbook supplies. Eventually, we buy glue, a jar of glitter, and a package of gold rickrack that Dad thinks will be ideal for circus costumes. Then we head out to Cracker Barrel where I wrap my fingers around a mug of coffee and watch Dad polish off a couple of biscuits with gravy.

"Mmmm . . . good," he says, rolling his eyes. "The best paste I ever ate."

On these short trips, time slows down. I sometimes feel as though I'm treating Dad like a child, indulging him in bags of sugary candies or sheets of stickers, but he doesn't seem to mind. At home, his anger flares up when he can't find his keys or his latest sketchpad. But things are good on these outings, where I have the luxury of saying yes to everything and letting him go at his own pace.

"Take the old road," Dad says as we leave Albuquerque.

I get off the interstate and cut down to Old 66 where we wind through Tijeras Canyon, past the big rocks that look like the voluptuous bodies of sleeping giantesses, and back up the road home.

Just like Dad, my mom never drives the freeway if she can help it, preferring to roll along the old two-lane highway as it twists and turns through the canyon into Albuquerque. One day, she and I take the slow road to Rowland Nursery to look for plants to fill the garden outside my French doors.

She picks up a small potted coleus. The plant's orange and burgundy leaves are so lush they look quilted and so richly colored I want to put my tongue on them. "Now is that beautiful or what?" she asks. Her brown eyes sparkle with excitement beneath the straight line of her bangs.

I like leaves more than flowers, especially oddly colored leaves. I seek out the deep plums and purples of heucheras and the acid green and gray of licorice plants. Mom slows her steps and I loosen my arm from around her, add the coleus to our wagon, and walk ahead, scanning the aisles.

I think it was their love of detail that brought my parents together. They both take such a profound interest in the world. At a certain point, though, their interests diverged. My mom is a gardener and an animal lover. She would be happiest in an almost primordial world where nothing ever changes. Dad is a builder. He sees a stick and immediately imagines how with a few thrusts of his carving knife it can be reborn as a mermaid. He wants to make a mark on the landscape where Mom so carefully treads.

"Snow in Summer," Mom says behind me. Her voice is bright as if she is greeting an old friend. "Pa always had that in his garden. You should get some."

She holds the pot out and the ruffled green and white leaves of the plant tremble on delicate stems.

The air inside the nursery is warm and moist, a strong contrast to the hot, dry winds outside. I can feel the inside of my nose loosen up and my pores sigh with relief. All around us is the damp scent of earth and verdant growth. After nearly a year in New Mexico, I am still homesick for the green of Los Angeles. I am craving the big, tropical leaves of Birds of Paradise and philodendrons. I want to transform my little garden into a lush oasis in the pines.

I add the plant to our cart and lace my fingers through Mom's, trying to be mindful of my pace. She is often the first person to pick out an Indian arrowhead from a sea of jagged rocks and gravel. She will pull her car to the side of the road to inspect an unfamiliar purple flower in the ditch or rescue an errant beetle from certain extinction on the blacktop. Now she walks slowly beside me, inspecting each plant, taking time to rub the velvety leaves of rose-scented geranium between her thumb and forefinger and inhale the perfume.

All this stopping and looking used to drive me crazy as a kid. I just wanted to get where we were going. It wasn't until after I returned home from college that I developed an appreciation for her measured pace, but still it was not a pace that could sustain me. When I am with her sometimes I feel like I'm pedaling slowly on a bicycle, struggling to keep myself balanced. Right now, La's habit of rushing forward is the only way for me to make it through.

Though they couldn't be less alike, I am lucky to have two moms: the one who spent thirty-six hours in labor before I was cut from her belly and handed over to the nuns in the small brick hospital where I was born and the one who wore a dress the color of jacaranda blossoms when she married Dad just before my twelfth birthday. They have both been such strong influences in my life that somehow even my body reflects equal parts of these women. I have the height and lean arms of my stepmother and the sturdy legs and curving hips of my mother. My hands are square and rough at the knuckles like my mother's hands, punished by years of gardening without gloves, and like La's, whose hands ache at the joints from the effort of turning cold clay into coffee cups and cereal bowls on a wheel.

It is not just my body that bears the imprint of these women. Thanks to my mother, I have the ability to identify plants and discern a raven from a crow (the raven is bigger and looks blue in the sun). From La, I get my drive to action, my need to fix things. These forces brought me to New Mexico.

Sometimes these two influences are at war. The shyness and insecurity I inherited from my mother battle it out daily with La's brave and often blind self-confidence. Guided by the force of her will, she is often able to muscle through situations that would terrify my mother. She is, for example, navigating the unknown territory of my father's illness while Mom stands at the edge of the forest and waits for someone to bring a map.

The strengths and shortcomings of my two mothers are tangled up with all that I have been given by Dad. Dad shares Mom's reverence for the beauty and uniqueness of the world, but his intense drive to create quickened his pace, kept his hand moving over canvases and sketchpads late into the night. That pace is slowing now, which trips up La and me. I have come home to be with him and share this time, and I want to follow Dad's meandering, but my responsibilities often lengthen my stride.

When I look in the mirror, I see Dad's green eyes staring back through mine. I see his long torso reflected in my own. If I cut my head open right now, would I also see a faint shadow of forgetting?

Our cart is brimming over with plants when I realize I need to get back up to Tinkertown. I've got to make dinner and set out Dad's nighttime medicine. I've got to water the nasturtiums in front of the museum and make sure that Wallace hasn't gotten in any fights with the raccoons under the house. There are a hundred things I have to do and they pull so hard against Mom's unhurried browsing that my voice comes out louder than I expected.

"I've got to go," I say.

"You always do," Mom replies.

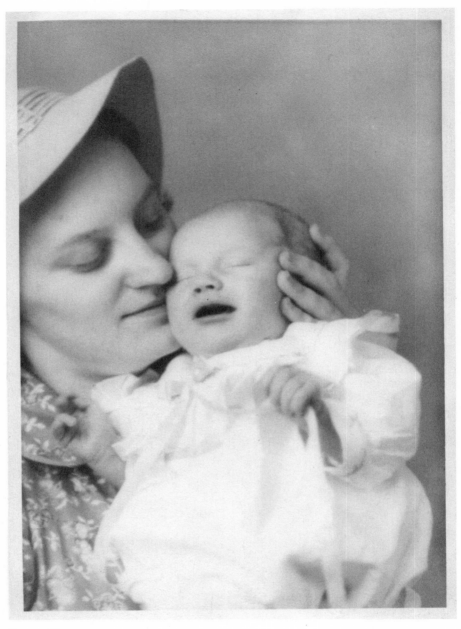

Rose and Ross 1940

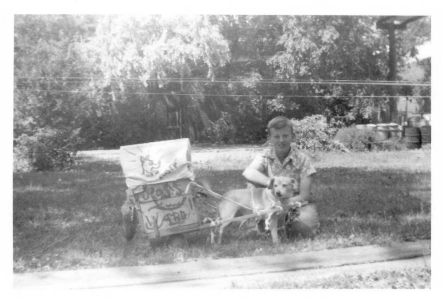

Ross and Rusty around 1952

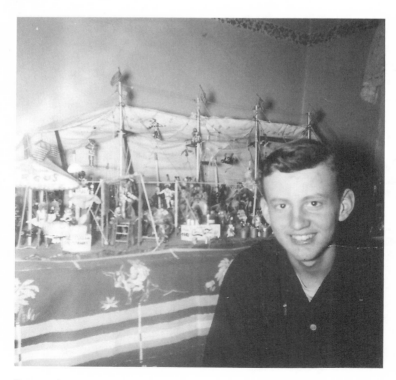

Ross 1956

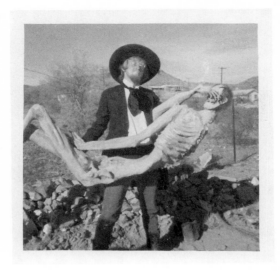

Ross 1966

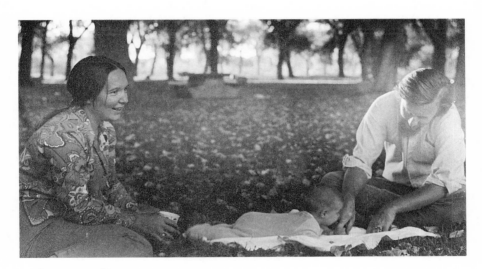

Sandra, Tanya, and Ross 1968

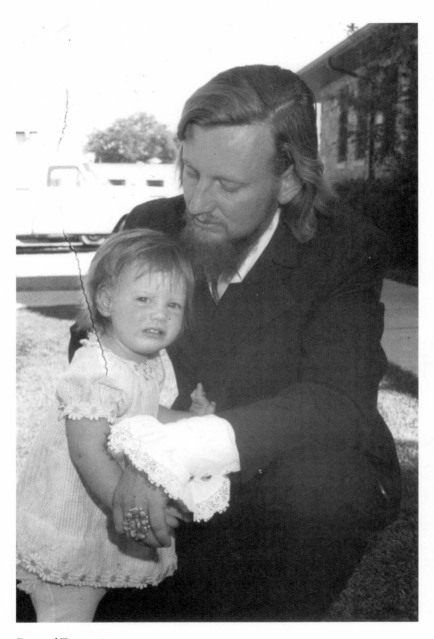

Ross and Tanya 1969

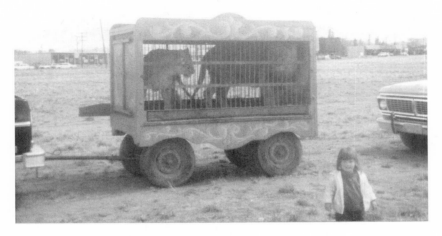

Tanya by the lions around 1970

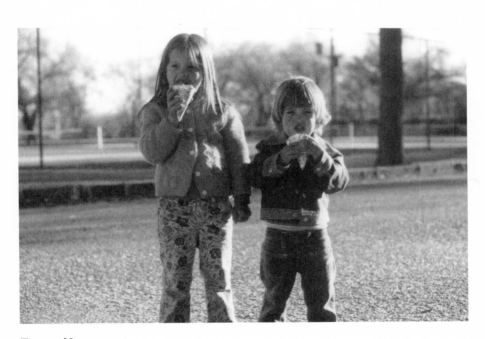

Tanya and Jason 1973

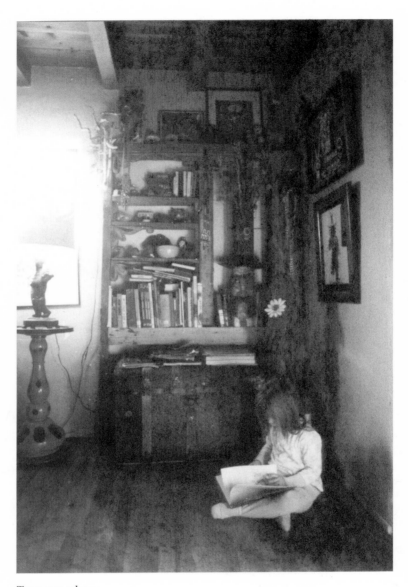

Tanya around 1974

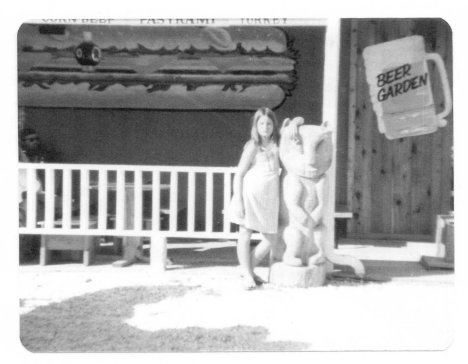

Tanya 1979

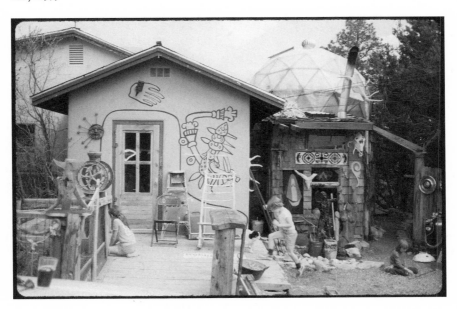

Our house 1977

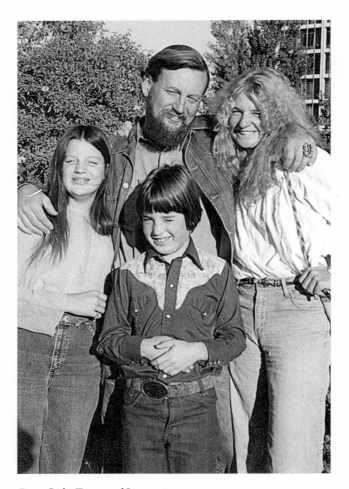

Ross, Carla, Tanya, and Jason 1982

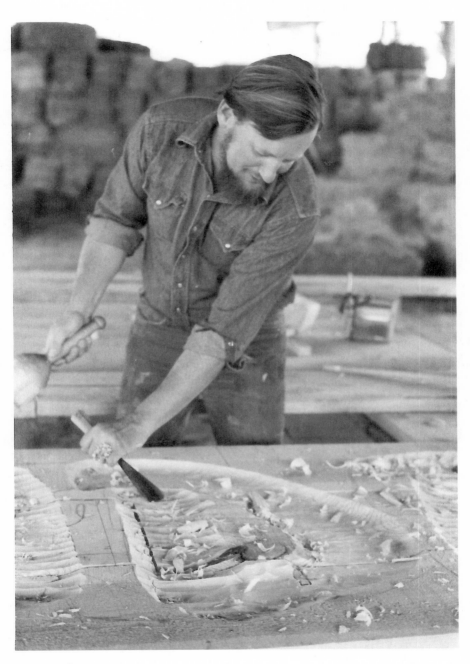

Ross around 1982

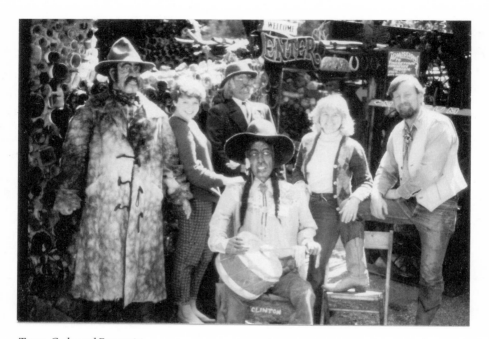

Tanya, Carla, and Ross 1986

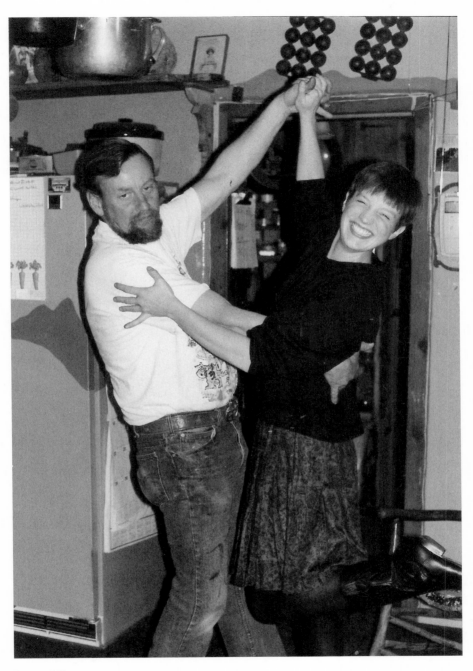

Ross and Tanya 1989

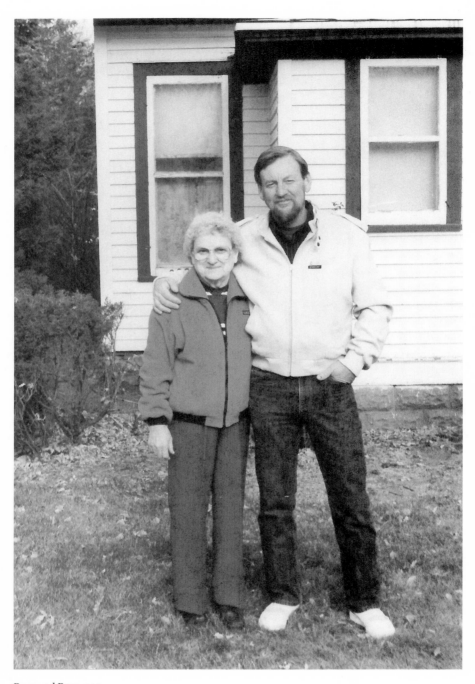

Rose and Ross 1990

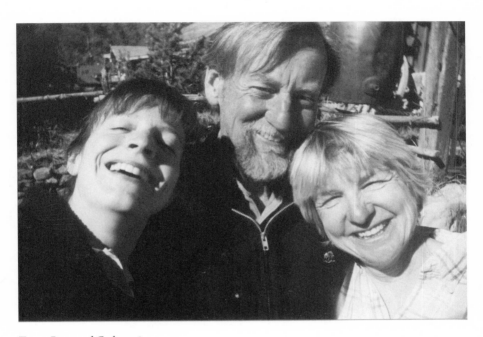

Tanya, Ross, and Carla 1998

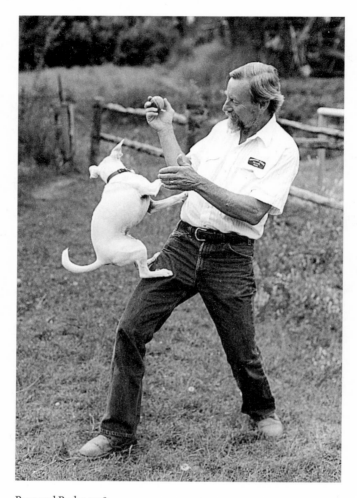

Ross and Radar 1998

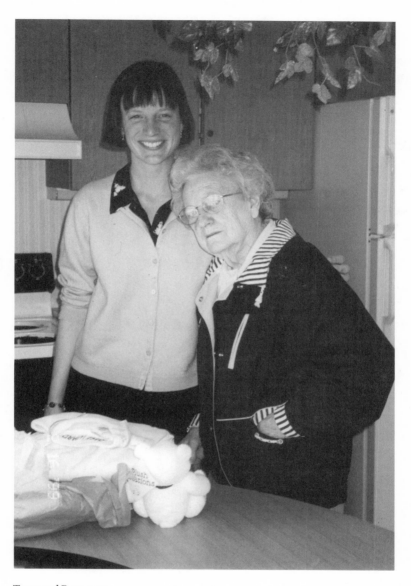

Tanya and Rose 1999

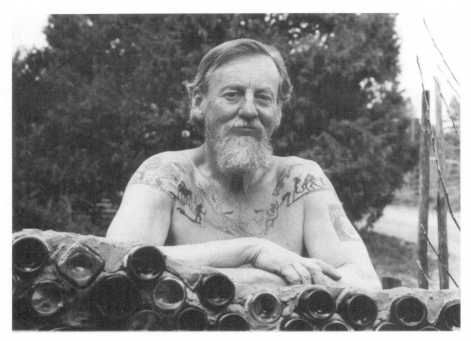

Ross 1999. PHOTO COURTESY OF STACY STUDEBAKER.

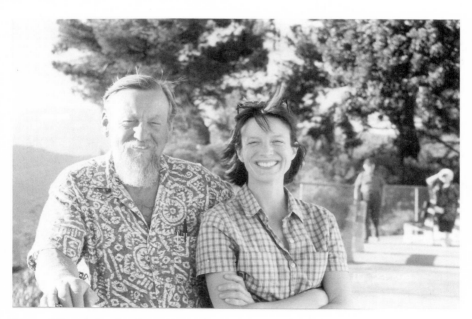

Ross and Tanya in Los Angeles 1999

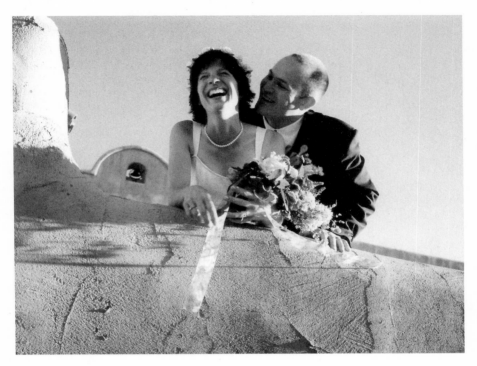

Tanya and David, June 16, 2001. PHOTO COURTESY OF KYLE ZIMMERMAN.

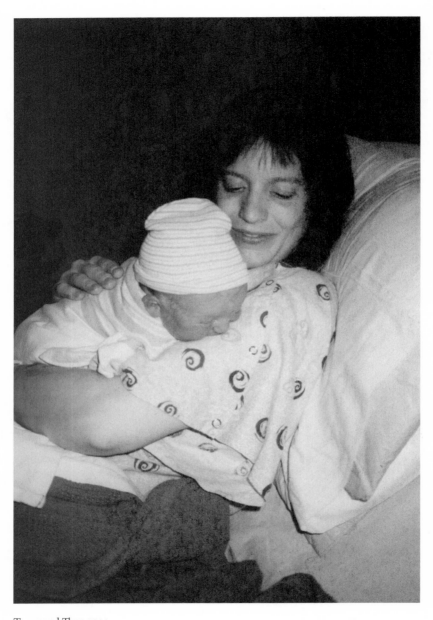

Tanya and Theo 2002

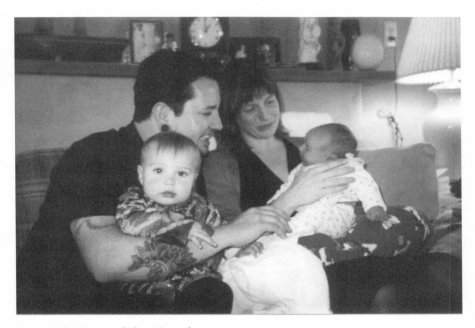

Jason, Hedy, Tanya, and Theo, November 2002

Bad Dreams and Brushfires ∗ *May 1999*

I AM ON MY BACK in my bed, staring up at the knotty pine beams of my bedroom ceiling and trying to breathe. A sharp pain wracks my chest. Each shallow breath intensifies the pain. I'm scared. For a minute I wonder if I'm dying. I wonder if I should call next door to the cottage and ask for help. My breathing quickens as though I am being chased.

When I was little—maybe seven or eight—I had what I called witch dreams. All around me I heard whispering, and although I strained my eyes to find the source of this sound, there was nothing but thick clouds and pale light. At the beginning, the clouds would move slowly and the whispers were so distant I couldn't be sure they were voices at all, but eventually, the rolling motion would quicken and the whispering would rise to the unintelligible cacophony of a flock of gulls. Bodies would emerge briefly from the clouds before disappearing just as quickly. When I woke from these dreams, I couldn't breathe. I couldn't cry. I could only wring my hands and pace the room, unable to soothe myself. It was not until I heard the loud click of the kitchen light switch and the even slap of Dad's leather slippers against the wood floors that my heartbeat would begin to slow.

"Hey there, squirt," he might say, brushing my hair out of my eyes with his big hands. "What's all the fuss?" He'd check under my bed and open the closet to look for monsters. He'd help me back into my bed and pull the covers up, tucking them tight all around my body. Then he would sit on the edge of my mattress and wait for my eyes to close. It was hard to go back to sleep, hard for my heart to let go of its fierce rhythm, but eventually, in the comforting presence of my dad, I would drift off.

Tonight, I try to imagine that Dad is here, holding my face between his wide palms, brushing my hair back, checking for monsters, but in the end, I open my eyes and look around my room. I am alone.

I focus on the only piece of Dad's art that I really consider mine—a pencil drawing called "Madame Alexander's Farewell." It is a drawing of a bubble. Just outside the bubble, his arm following its curve, is Dad. He kneels before a young woman dressed in striped bell-bottom trousers. She is me, or at least a vision Dad had of me. My long hair flows down my back. I have one hand on a door handle and the other held palm up to receive a key Dad offers. Inside the bubble are my dolls and a wind-up apple I played with as a child. Beyond the door are rocks, rough waves, and cactus; and, in the far distance, the empty chair Dad often uses to symbolize death. In this drawing Dad seems to bow to my inevitable departure. My eyes are clear and bright. Inside Dad's head is the shadowy face of an old man.

Dad often drew or painted my mother and, later, La, but with the exception of silly cartoons, he had never before turned his creativity loose on me. I immediately assumed ownership of this drawing and wrote out a "sold" sign that I tucked into the frame when it was displayed at arts and crafts fairs and galleries.

"Oh, I'd let it go for about five bucks," Dad used to joke. "Some guy comes in here with two bits and he's taking that thing home."

"It's not for sale," I would declare primly. "It's mine."

"If you say so, Daughter." Dad would laugh.

Three years ago, Dad finally gave me the drawing. On the back, he scrawled "Madame Alexander finally gets on the road after 18 years! Love Ross (Daddy)." I drove it back to Los Angeles and hung it in the big house I shared with my successful lawyer boyfriend. I felt like I had left the bubble. I had no idea that I would be back here in my old bedroom with the drawing hanging opposite my bed as though nothing had changed.

The phone rings. The sound pulls me from sleep like a fish on a line. I am up, on the surface, gasping for air.

"Hello?"

There's a woman on the other end of the line. She wants to know when the museum opens, what's in it, and how much it will cost to see it. I mumble through my answers and wait for her to register the fact that it's so fucking early that I must actually live in the museum. But she doesn't. The phone rings at all hours and I shouldn't answer it, but how can it be helped that the number I give my friends and David is the same number printed on ten thousand four-color brochures distributed throughout the state? When you live in a museum, you are part of the museum.

When I have satisfied the curiosity of the woman on the phone, I lean back into the sheets and try to work myself back into sleep, but all that comes is the recollection of that terrible, pinching feeling in my chest. I think about it cautiously, the way you flex a foot after a bad cramp and find that the pain is still there, waiting. I don't have to Google "anxiety attack" to have a pretty good idea of what's happening to me.

A couple of months ago, we saw smoke in the backyard. When we ran out with the hose to douse the flames, we realized that the ground was hot in dozens of spots. We started digging and found that Dad had been burying the ashes from the stove without making sure they were cold. The layer of dirt kept the embers alive, and when we dug into the holes, the burst of air ignited tiny flames. La grabbed a bucket and another shovel and we turned over the entire yard, dousing it with water. The mud steamed and sizzled and the air smelled of burnt grass.

I think about these fires now. It's as if someone has taken a shovel and knocked open the cage of my chest and fanned the flames of my panic until I'm not sure they will ever be put out.

At dinner with Mom, I say, "I hate this place. I hate it." I can feel my face flush. I hate that Dad is sick and that I'm running out of money and that my boyfriend lives in another state. I hate that I'm not writing.

And she says, "Then leave. Go back to Los Angeles. Have a life, Tanya. Don't stay here for us."

"But I can't," I say.

"Why not?"

"I can't leave. I don't want to disappoint everyone."

"Then you risk disappointing yourself."

I should be happy to hear this, but it only makes me mad. I know she speaks from experience. She spent years standing in the shadow of my father's career, watching him cheat on her with other women. When, after the divorce, she remarried, it was to another artist and as his wife she drifted back into familiar shadows. He beat her and shouted at her and one day killed three of her chickens with a two-by-four.

When, at last, that marriage ended, she got involved with a Volvo mechanic who'd fought a lifelong battle with depression and alcoholism. After the mechanic, there was the waiter with four children and a cocaine habit. He moved on, but Mom had sustained a bruise to the heart and soul that would take a long time to heal. I've tried to save my share of cute boys with addictive personalities, so I know where she's coming from, but I can't take her advice.

"I don't think I could do what you're doing, Tanya," Mom says.

This is true. She can't enter a hospital room. She will listen wide-eyed to my descriptions of Grandma with poop in her pants, but she won't visit her. I wish I didn't have to do these things, but I can't keep from doing them. I am angry with Mom because she is saying out loud exactly what I think. What is keeping me here?

Years ago, when I joined my dad and my uncle Louie on a carnival road trip, we called ourselves "Pop, Punk, and Unk." I helped roll out primer on the metal panels of the sled ride known as a "Flying Bobs" and carefully colored in Dad's outlines of cotton-candy clouds or caramel apples. Sometimes I made us lunches of peanut butter and jelly sandwiches, the jam spread so thick, a crimson ooze marked each bite. On one of these trips, I rested on the bed in the back of the van while Dad drove out toward Knott's Berry Farm. The streetlights along I-5 were flickering to life as I heard Dad tell Louie he was glad to have me along. "If it weren't for the kid, here, we'd probably spend the night in some bar, but instead we're off to Knott's. Now that's something."

I liked hearing this. I liked knowing that I was making a difference just by being there. I feel like I'm making a difference now and as hard as it is to stay, I don't think it's time to leave.

A Hell of a Time * May 1999

"I HAVE AN APPOINTMENT with a therapist," I tell La. I say this fast so that maybe she won't hear. She is hanging a collection of Dad's etchings on the wall. She puts down her hammer and turns to me.

"This is a hard time," La says. She puts an arm around my shoulder and leans against me. I stand very quietly, the way you would if a wild animal suddenly nuzzled your hand for food. I don't want to startle her out of this moment, but then the phone on her belt rings and she is walking away with the receiver pressed to her ear.

The therapist's name is Johanna. I met her at a women's creativity conference in Albuquerque, where she sat in a booth and offered flyers on depression and anxiety along with paper cups of herb tea. She had a low, kind voice and a level gaze, and she listened carefully when I explained what had been happening since my move home. I could feel my throat tighten and my eyes begin to prickle with tears as I gratefully accepted her business card. I resisted the urge to throw myself, weeping, into her lap.

Maybe to counteract her first impression of me, I have dressed carefully for my appointment. I skip my baggy overalls in favor of a tomato-colored, sleeveless linen dress and black sandals. I slip on earrings and a silver bracelet. I brush my hair and swipe mascara onto my lashes. I make a careful appraisal in the mirror and decide that I look grown up and in charge. I need help, but I am not helpless.

Johanna is a small woman with short, gray hair and square, plastic spectacles. Along with her woven tunic, she wears clogs and a necklace made of several stone amulets. The spiral logo that is on her business card is a theme in her office, gracing the throw on the couch and duplicated in metal sculpture over her desk. She follows my eyes to the spiral.

"It's a maze," she says. "The journey inward."

I want to say, "duh," but I need her help more than I need to be sarcastic.

Johanna is the fifth therapist I have seen since college. I feel that by now I should have a pamphlet summary of my life that I can hand out at these inaugural meetings. But instead, I know I will sit for the first hour and explain my parents' divorce, my dad's illness, the museum, the carnival, and the way I both fit and don't fit in my family. The fact that I've been to as many therapists as I have is one of the ways that I don't fit. Talking to a stranger about my feelings does not fall under the heading of "the show must go on." I wonder if I'll get credit for facing my danger if I do so with a therapist's help.

About ten minutes into this first session, my mascara is running down my cheeks and my nervous hands have crumpled the lap of my linen dress. I am acutely aware of the stale funk of sadness and fear drifting up from my armpits. I explain about the panic attacks, the wild fluttering of wings in my chest, the sharp pain that makes even the slightest inhalation feel like a stab wound. I explain how a broken copy machine can trigger an hour of weeping, how it has become harder and harder to get dressed. There are days when I want to rip the clothes from my body. I feel constricted and constrained, agitated by the touch of fabric to skin. I cry so much, the shape of my mouth feels swollen and unfamiliar, as though it will never shut properly again. We go over the fifty-minute hour by nearly forty minutes, but she doesn't charge me for the extra time. Instead, she gives me a bottle with a blue and white label. Inside are five pills.

"Start with half of one," she says. "We might have to fiddle with it at first, but we'll figure out a way for it to work. You were right to ask for help."

I slip the bottle into my purse. On the way home, I can almost feel the vibrations of the capsules on the seat beside me. I feel awkward about going on medication. I wonder what La will say.

Back at home, I walk down the driveway, knowing my red eyes match the color of my dress. I am hoping to get into the house where I can splash water on my face and brush my hair before I have to talk to anyone, but La springs out of the gift shop and meets me halfway.

"How'd it go?" she asks.

"She put me on antidepressants," I say. I feel my mouth tighten with embarrassment, but I will the words out anyway. I wait for La to judge my weakness. I wait for her to tell me to toughen up.

"I'm taking Wellbutrin," La says. "I feel a little better. Your dad's on something too. What's she got you on?"

It surprises me that La could have slowed down enough to ask for help.

"I've got to get back in the shop," she says, giving me a quick squeeze. "We've got a school group in the back and things are about to get rowdy."

"Do you need help?" I ask.

"Take a break," she says. "Get your bearings."

I am on Zoloft. Dad is taking Klonopin. La is taking Wellbutrin. At Manor Care, Grandma swallows a handful of pills from a white paper cup without asking any questions.

On the kitchen counter in the cottage are two pillboxes labeled with the days of the week. La labels them "AM" and "PM" with a Sharpie and at breakfast and dinner Dad grabs the contents in grumpy handfuls from the placemat and swallows them without water. Sometimes he chews them up. I can't help but grimace. Mixed in with the prescriptions are big amber-colored capsules of vitamin E, which thins his blood so every time he picks at a scab or the corner of a fingernail, he bleeds and bleeds and bleeds.

"Take care of yourself," the therapist says. "Be nicer to yourself."

David says this too. I close my eyes and try to see that happy girl on the videotape, the one with the calm eyes and easy smile. But it's hard to find her in the angry person who throws a box of brochures across the room because they won't fold or tears all the buttons off a blouse because it feels so constricting against her skin. I feel suffocated by the darkness in the Tinkertown house. I feel my own place in the world dissolving in the tide of Dad's forgetting.

Rock Runs * *August 1999*

BECAUSE THE AD AGENCY isn't generating enough profit to pay all of us, I've stopped going in every day. Megan does the bulk of the design and I show up once a week to pound out some copy and take Megan to lunch. The rest of the time I spend opening the museum, working shifts in the gift shop and following Dad from room to room in the house to make sure he doesn't take his clothes off and pee in the yard or walk down to the Shell station for a six-pack of beer. I miss Megan's company, our mornings on the front steps, and even our self-imposed nine-to-five schedule. My time now has taken a much looser form.

Most days we head out on what Dad calls a "rock run." We drive up the road from our house into the Cibola National Forest or head out along North 14 up toward the tiny coal-mining town of Madrid where the rounded hills are dotted like Dalmatians with piñon trees. Today we are less than a mile from Tinkertown on a hillside of deep red rock and sliding gravel when Dad shouts, "There's a beauty!"

He jumps out of the car and scrambles up the side of the hill, which falls away under his heels. Pebbles bounce and skitter to the asphalt as he begins to struggle with a rock roughly the size of my torso. He muscles it out of the ground and starts rolling it down the hill. Other rocks are dislodged as this mammoth thing rolls past, and I have a very clear image of it crashing into the side of the car. Dad hoots with laughter.

Together we heft the huge rock up into the trunk where it joins half a dozen others. My Honda sags under the weight, and I lean in and look up into the wheel well above the tire. Metal is nearly touching rubber— always the signal that it is time to go home.

"But what about that one?" Dad asks, pointing to another behemoth.

"Next time."

We unload the rocks in the backyard of the cottage where they join hundreds more. Since my move home, Dad has rearranged these rocks almost daily into two long trails that snake across the yard and catch La off guard as she stomps off to feed the horses or runs to answer the phone. I have stubbed my toe on them a dozen times, but it doesn't keep Dad from moving the rocks again and again, shifting the two lines to form a different open-ended trail leading off into the forest.

When we're tired of hauling stuff, Dad and I mix up a tub of cement and he works on the bottle walls he's begun outside the cottage window. I make sure he doesn't add too much water to the mud, and I hand him bottles from a pile. Every few minutes he steps back to admire his handiwork.

I remember once how he gave me a lesson in wall building. He showed me how to dig a trench and fill it with wire and rocks and cement.

"Then you stick these guys in," he said, handing me a few lengths of rebar. "To give it a backbone."

When the rebar was set, he carefully laid a row of rock and then a row of bottles, all the time winding baling wire through the whole thing for added strength.

"Look at this," he said, holding a tangle of wire. "Free building material. All you got to do is buy a truckload of hay. Guess those horses are worth something after all."

He dug in his shirt pocket for a piece of paper, drew a quick "builder's plan," and handed it to me.

"Now, you'll never have to live in a tent."

These new walls are not as sturdy. We've skipped the foundation and left out the rebar and wire. But it doesn't matter. Each night, before the cement fully sets, La and I take down the walls a few rows at a time.

"It's a good project," La says. "But I can't stand to lose the sunlight."

Dad doesn't notice that the walls never grow; he's just having a good time building them.

I lose myself in this kind of physical activity. Working side by side with Dad I don't have to think about how his words are drifting away, light and fine as dust in the breeze. Even old standbys like "fork" and "cup" are as elusive as five-dollar words like "cacophony" or "metamorphosis." I like the word "wilderness." I like "fishnet" and "harmony" and "butterbean." They sound beautiful. Words like "symphony" and "heliport" and "olallieberry" sit on my tongue like rare sweets. Losing words for me would be like losing my ability to taste.

The work takes my mind off my life too. Or lack of it. I'm starting to identify with those walls—building up during the day and then shrinking back down at night. Perpetually in an unfinished state. Though I've started a screenplay and a few short stories and had great hopes of making a documentary about Dad, I haven't really pursued any of these things. At night, if I'm not watching television with Dad and La, I'm asleep by nine in the Tinkertown house. I miss David all the time.

When I first moved home, Dad asked over and over, "What are you doing here, again? I thought you lived in Los Angeles." He's stopped asking, but I haven't stopped thinking about it.

In the last couple of months, La has been asking more about David. She's stopped calling him my "little friend" and started wondering what kind of plans we have for the future.

"I don't know," I say.

"You can't make plans for the future right now, anyway," she says.

I wonder if she's confusing her future with mine. Her certainty makes me angry. I don't want to spend the rest of my life in the dark, crowded Tinkertown house. I feel more and more that it's time to start shaping my own destiny. I want to go back to Los Angeles and marry David and start my own family, but I've been too scared to say it out loud. It's time for that to change.

Homecoming ✳ *September 1999*

WHEN I ASK IF I can move into his apartment in Los Angles, David lets out a whoop of joy so loud I have to hold the phone away from my ear.

"You're not joking, are you?" he says.

"No," I say. "But if you think I should get my own place, I'll understand."

"When are you coming?" he asks.

I haven't really stopped to think about the logistics. David is the first person I've told of my decision. Although this makes sense, it feels odd and unfamiliar to leave my family out.

"I'm not sure," I say. "As soon as I can."

A few hours later, La and I are sitting on the back porch of the Tinkertown house. Hummingbirds helicopter around our heads, and Otto the band organ in the museum shudders to life, ripping out a military march with plenty of drums.

"I want to go back to Los Angeles," I say.

La looks right into my face.

"Where will you live?"

"With David."

"Does he want to marry you?" she asks.

"I think he does," I say. This is the first time I have said it out loud, and because it is the first time it seems fragile and precious and makes my cheeks burn with the reality of my decision.

"Well, you could do worse," she says.

When David and I first met I was in the throes of a breakup. I was looking for an apartment and packing and crying a lot. In the midst of all of this, I spent a bit of time musing about a previous boyfriend. I thought the English musician with a face like a lion might have been the right one. Maybe I'd made a wrong turn when I moved in with the lawyer. I wondered aloud about this with David one day while we were working and he looked up from the computer screen and offered to track the guy down. In that moment, our relationship changed. Later, after we'd kissed, I asked David why he would want to search out my old boyfriend when he himself had designs on me.

"More than anything," he said, "I wanted you to be happy."

I want La to be happier for me. I want her to celebrate my decision. I have found the person with whom I want to spend my life. La reaches out and gives my elbow a little squeeze.

"When do you think you'll go?" she asks, moving past emotion to logistics.

"I'm really happy," I say. I'm being petulant because I can't just come out and ask her to be happy for me.

"Of course you are, but things don't just stop around here because you're leaving," she says.

"I'm not asking everything to stop. Just pause. Everything always has to be so huge with you," I say.

"I fucking love you, Tanya," La says. "I do. I'm going to miss the hell out of you. But I need to make plans. When do you think you'll leave?"

I am forgetting the credo: The show must go on. "Whenever is convenient," I say. "I don't want to leave you in the lurch."

La reminds me that she has a big horse show coming up, and I promise to stay until after it ends.

"What about Christmas?" she asks. "Would you stay for the holidays?"

She does not have to say that we have a finite number of holidays left with my father. Although it means delaying my move by nearly three months, I agree not to leave until after the New Year.

La has the ability to make me angrier than any person on the planet. She is speedy and sloppy and sometimes thoughtless. Her self-reliance can sometimes feel bossy and selfish. But she is also the person who gave me three pairs of Guess Jeans in 1985 when those things were like gold in the social stock market of high school. She is the person who sent me a copy of *Writer's Market* when I showed her my first piece of college creative writing. She is the one other person who loves my dad as much as I do. There are those who believe that we "choose" our parents. I feel grateful that I chose one extra who so completely challenges and supports me. Sometimes she is the danger, but more often, she is right there beside me as we face it together.

"So, are we okay?" La asks.

"Yes," I say. And I mean it.

Pedal to the Metal Back to Los Angeles
✳ *October 1999*

I'VE GOT THE RADIO cranked up, the windows down, and Dad and I are singing along with Patsy Cline as we blaze through Albuquerque, following I-40 West. We are leaving the piles of icy, white, early snow and going as far as the Pacific Ocean. I have cleared out my Tinkertown "suite," and the big green chair sits in the back of La's pickup surrounded by boxes of books, clothes, bedding, and a big box of pots and pans. I can't help but smile at the thought of cooking with David and dancing together on the red-and-plum-colored tile of his tiny kitchen.

I look across at Dad, and he flashes me a big smile. "We stole this darned truck," he says gleefully. "Go, go, go," he roars.

I laugh and tell him I'm going as fast as I can. I am still surprised that he agreed to join me. In the past months, it's been harder and harder to get him off the sofa even for a short trip to the hardware store. In the days before our departure, I prepared him the way a mother prepares a child for a new experience, trusting that repetition will breed familiarity and comfort. We talked of roller coasters and Hollywood and the sandy beaches of Malibu. I'm not sure how much he understands, but I know that this is our last road trip together. I plan to do everything in my power to make it a good one.

It is nearly eight o' clock when we take the truck up the steep hill of Baxter Street and stop in front of the Echo Park duplex I will share with David. David rushes down the stairs to hug me and shake Dad's hand.

"I can't believe you're here," he says. "Wow, you've got a lot of stuff."

"Your future is filled with my stuff," I say.

"Well, let's unload and get going," David says. He kisses me and grabs a box and leads the way up the stairs.

It is night and I am in bed next to David. It took a while to help Dad understand that we weren't going to go right back home. We called La to let her know we had arrived, and she reassured Dad that it would be only a few days. I made up a bed for him in David's office and left the bathroom light on so he'd be sure to find his way. Tomorrow, while David is at work, Dad and I will head out to the beach, but right now, I rest my palm on the warm skin of David's chest and align my breath with his.

The next day it's eighty degrees, and with the sun blazing across the sparkling blue of the Pacific and glinting on the white sand, the snowy mountains of New Mexico are a swiftly receding memory. Dad stares out at the sea. He's unbuttoned the first couple of buttons on his Hawaiian shirt, and his long, gray beard blows in the breeze. With one thick forefinger, he draws squiggles in the sand next to him. He looks calm and happy. I pull out my camera and focus on his hand in the sand and snap the shutter. He looks up and sticks his tongue out, rolling his eyes.

"Yes, my child," he says.

I take another photo. I take pictures of his hands and the deep laugh lines around his eyes. I snap the shutter on the way his hair curves up at the base of his neck and the cracked skin of his knuckles. I suddenly feel compelled to document every part of him, to commit to film the way his back curves and his feet splay out in the sand. I want photographs of his wide, meaty palms and his pale eyelashes and the sliver of gold filling in his front tooth. I snap the shutter again and again until he begins to ignore me, until I finally run out of film. I don't want to trust these precious parts to my own flimsy memory. I want them printed out on paper. I want something I can touch when Dad is no longer with me.

I wake the next morning to find Dad dressed and sitting on the couch.

"You got a minute?" he says. He leads me into the office, where he's filled the big dry erase board with drawings. He's aged himself, making his beard even longer, and drawn me in my overall shorts, my hair in a neat bob. "On to Knotts," the board reads. Under the figure of me is scrawled, "dear, darling child of the West."

"Wow," I say.

"I guess the old man can still draw," Dad says. He is flushed with pride, his eyes sparkling.

"I guess you're ready to go to Knott's Berry Farm," I say.

"Hell yes, Daughter," Dad says.

The black-and-white photograph commemorating Dad's first visit to Knott's Berry Farm shows a nine-year-old boy in a plaid shirt and jeans with wide-rolled cuffs astride a stuffed bucking horse. The photo was taken in 1949, when Knott's was still a functioning berry farm with a restaurant serving chicken and biscuits. There were no rides, just an old western town and a museum of miniatures. This visit crystallized Dad's vision of his future. From that time on, he never had a doubt about what he wanted. He wanted a place like Knott's.

When Dad, David, and I arrive at Knott's Berry Farm, I take a careful look at the map. I want to stick to the few areas that are just as Dad remembers. The only new thing that cannot be avoided is the enormous wooden coaster known as the Ghostrider. Dad has been pining after this coaster like a kid since we hit the road in Albuquerque.

"Are you ready?" Dad asks in his best midway voice. "Are you ready to go fast?"

I get in the front with Dad behind me. David takes the next car. I can feel my heart beating as we click, click, click up the first steep hill. I hear screams from ahead as the train in front crests the top and zooms down the other side. The cross bars shift and creak like a boat and click beneath the rails. I don't like feeling trapped and out of control, but I realize once we make this slow climb, there is no escaping the inevitable drop. I think of Dad's diagnosis and how that has changed my life. I think of the five-year timeline set by the doctors, more than two years of which have already passed.

At the top, the car pauses for a moment, and I look out ahead at the long curving track. I can feel the warmth of Dad's body at my back. All I can do is hold on tight and try to have a good time.

That night, in the living room of the apartment, I tell Dad that I'm going to marry David. I'm jumping the gun here. David hasn't actually asked me and I have no idea when he will, but I can't be sure how present Dad will be in a month or a year and so I want to take this moment to tell him that I've found my match.

Dad gives me a wink. "Well, Daughter, I don't see anything wrong with that."

Late the next morning I fasten Dad's seatbelt and turn to give David a fierce hug. Though I will miss him, this parting is not nearly as hard as all of those that have come before. I practically live here now.

"*Adios*, pardner," Dad shouts. "*Vaya con dios*, etcetera, etcetera . . ."

It is near dark when we arrive in Flagstaff, and Dad's sunny mood left long before the actual sun set. He's tired and hungry and confused.

"Does Carla know you have her truck?" he asks. "What are we doing out here?"

I try to calm him down, assuring him that we will stay overnight here and leave first thing in the morning.

"We'll be home for lunch," I say cheerily, hoping to buoy him.

"Fuck lunch," he says.

I steer the truck into the first motel I see. The windows of the office give off a flickering white light—a mix of fluorescents and television. The place is little more than a strip of doors facing the highway.

Inside, it isn't much more appealing. The beds are sagging, the chipped Formica dresser is missing a couple of drawer pulls and there's a big rust stain running down the side of the sink like an old wound. Dad sits on the edge of the bed and rubs his eyes while I head into the bathroom. I am sitting on the toilet with my jeans around my ankles when I hear the front door of our room open and close. I am up like a shot, still buttoning my jeans when I pull open the door to see Dad halfway across the parking lot.

"Hey," I shout. "Dad?" I can hear the panic in my voice and I try to take a deep breath while simultaneously sprinting over to him.

"Where you headed?" I ask. This time, I will my voice to be calm.

"Home, I guess," Dad says.

"For tonight, home is here," I say gesturing expansively at the junky hotel.

"Bullshit," he says, but he lets me take his arm and lead him back into our room and help him into bed.

When I hear Dad begin to snore from the bed next to mine, I climb out of the stiff, scratchy sheets and push the dresser in front of the door. On my way back to bed, I stop and take a long look at Dad. He's curled on his side, his hair falling over his forehead. He's left a big space on the right side of the bed. This space is for La. In all the months I've slept in the Tinkertown house, I've left a similar space for David. Halfway between Albuquerque and Los Angeles, this funky hotel room standing in for limbo, I know that moving back to Los Angeles is the right decision.

Christmas 1999

MY MOM IS SITTING next to La and they are laughing at some shared joke. We are celebrating with Megan's parents, Bruce and Doreen. Although they split up a couple of years ago, they remain good friends and continue to share a meal several times a week. I think this might be the true meaning of Christmas.

My family's support of my move is evident with every gift. I receive a "Do Not Disturb" sign, a jar of relaxing bath salts, a satin eye pillow, and a book on meditation.

"Am I a little tightly wound?" I ask. "It's not like my time here was stressful or anything . . ."

From Megan and Jason comes a silver corkscrew shaped like a frog. The card reads "Fear not! Taking a leap (of faith) will open up something quite delicious."

I give Megan a pair of earrings and a card with a photo of the two of us sitting on the stoop in the blazing New Mexico sunshine. Megan pulls me into a hug.

"Hey, there, you two," Jason says. He purses his lips and blows us a kiss before snapping a picture. The dogs start to wrestle and growl in the piles of crumpled paper and Megan and I pull apart and wipe our eyes.

We are so caught up that we don't notice that Dad has disappeared. When La finds him in the kitchen, he has a bottle of vodka to his lips, drinking it in quick gulps like water. Our holiday is over.

We move quickly to get Dad into his coat and into the truck. Though it's a forty-minute drive from Bruce's house in Albuquerque up to Tinkertown, La assures us that she'll be fine driving him home as long as I follow right behind in my car.

"It doesn't make sense to leave a car," she says. "Besides, he's just going to pass out."

I rush to pack up things and grab my own coat and boots. Mom follows me, her brows knitting together in a worried line.

"What can I do?" she asks. "This is just awful."

"It is awful," I say. "But he doesn't know what he's doing."

"He was sad tonight," she says. "I thought something like this would happen."

I think back to earlier, when Dad was holding a string of ribbons and making Radar jump in the air. He was laughing.

"I don't think he was sad," I say. "I think he saw an opportunity and took it. He just doesn't remember how much is too much."

"Well, I don't know," Mom says. "I just feel bad for Carla and for you. You shouldn't have to do this."

The air is cold and crisp and filled with the scent of wood smoke. I hug Mom and promise to call her in the morning. I need to get going if I'm going to catch up with La. I don't want her to have to do this alone.

The lights in the cabin are ablaze when I drive through the gates of Tinkertown and La runs out, still in her coat, to greet me.

"Your dad's in the truck. I hope he's not frozen to death," she says. "He jumped out on the way home. I was slowing down for a light, but I think he has a black eye."

La has tucked a sleeping bag around Dad. He's snoring, but the truck is already getting cold and there is no way we can leave him here.

"Honey," La says, "let's go." She clicks her tongue the way she would to get a horse to move, and Dad stirs.

We manage to drag him out of the truck and then we are stumbling through the snow, our bodies buckling under the weight of my father. Dad's eyes open for a moment and he mumbles something and leans in as though to kiss me. I can smell his breath, as hot and eye-watering as kerosene.

"Hey, it's me, Dad," I say. "It's Tanya."

He pulls back and closes his eyes. This is the first time I have not been angry about Dad's drinking. They say that alcoholism is a disease, but it's no match for Alzheimer's. I know the craving is hardwired, but I always felt that Dad could stop if he wanted. When he decided to drink instead of spending time with me, I felt angry and hurt. Now, there are no decisions to be made. The plaques and tangles are closing in, strangling willpower and independent thought. All this time, we've been saying that Dad is battling Alzheimer's. We've said it so much that I can close my eyes and see him, sword aloft, fending off the huge snake of forgetting. Tonight, I can see that no matter how strong he is, it's still a losing battle. I am not angry, but I am sad clear through.

We lug him up the steps and down the walk to the front door, past the kitchen table, and into the bedroom where we dump him on the bed and stop to catch our breath.

"Well, shit," La says. "Merry Christmas."

A New Year * *January 2000*

DAVID AND I HAVE SPENT the whole day in the kitchen of the Tinkertown house, getting ready to feed practically everyone I know. He's cutting onions because with his contact lenses in, he doesn't cry. I am peeling a mountain of potatoes. We've got a turkey in the oven, a big pot of caramelized leek gravy bubbling on the stove, and mussels on ice waiting for a last-minute steam bath of white wine, garlic, and herbs.

The television news is filled with predictions and postulations about that minute past midnight leading into a year filled with zeros. How will the clocks work, they wonder? How will the computers keep time? I think of Dad and his wish to be fused with La in the melted glass of the museum after a nuclear blast. I understand where that comes from. Tonight, we'll have lots of champagne in the fridge, the people we love all around us, and if the world ends, then so be it.

Dad still has a bit of a black eye from his Christmas night tumble. He is slower and more tentative too, as though the battle of that night has left lasting scars. The changes in Dad seem to happen in chunks, less like his brain is being whittled away and more like someone sawed a piece right out. It's taking all of us time to get used to this new version of Dad. Though he doesn't say it, I think he's finding this latest change particularly uncomfortable. He sits in the kitchen rocker with his hands folded over his stomach and watches as David and I cook. Despite the heat of the oven, he is wearing the black down jacket that La gave him for Christmas zippered to his chin and a purple Tinkertown Museum cap pulled down over his eyes.

I hear the jingle of the wrought-iron door handle and the slam of the screen door followed by the thump, thump as La stamps snow off her boots.

"Smells great in here." She kneels in front of Dad. "Hey, honey, hey," she says. "You wanna get dressed for the party?"

"Party?" Dad asks.

"It's New Year's Eve," La says. "I'm gonna need a kiss at midnight from my sweetie."

"I've always got a kiss for my sweetheart," Dad says.

I think, no matter how much of Dad's brain goes away, the part that loves La will remain a green and living island in a dark sea of forgetting. I look at David. He's got a dishtowel over his shoulder and a growing pile of onions on the cutting board in front of him. I hope we can love each other as much.

I've set up the video camera on a tripod in my office and am urging everyone at the party to record something for posterity. Some, like my friend Nilz, whom I have known since second grade, need no urging. He clicks on the camera and speaks for some minutes in the "ubby dubby" language we learned years ago on the public television program Zoom. He dons bright pink "2000" glasses and cavorts wildly in front of the lens. My friend Brian eats a plate of turkey with gravy in front of the camera, savoring each bite. He wishes me happy cooking. He celebrates the fact that David and I will once again share a kitchen. My friend Brad is so tall, he has to slump down in the chair to fit in the frame. He wonders what he should say and stares into the camera with his brow furrowed in concentration. The cat, Pokey, jumps up onto his lap triggering a fit of sneezing. "Hello, cat, I'm so allergic to you . . . ," Brad says. He points the remote at the camera, trying in vain to turn it off.

I have known these three men since they were all boys. I crushed hard on all of them until, at some point, they took me out to dinner and came out of the closet for dessert. We have spent nearly every New Year's Eve of the past ten years together. I am glad they can join us here tonight; glad they can witness me on the cusp of change.

A fire crackles in the fireplace and candles wink across the mantel. Winter coats pile up on my bed as more people arrive. Kent, a self-proclaimed "mountain man" in a hand-stitched calico shirt and leather breeches, gives me a rib-crushing hug. "I'm not kidding, gal," he says. "Get you a life preserver out there in California and keep it close. One day you're gonna wash up on the shores of Arizona."

Florence and Maggie arrive together. "Yep," Florence says, "the two nuts . . ."

"Mutt and Jeff," Maggie echoes. "We're really gonna miss you, and how."

My eyes tear up.

"Well, don't get all weepy on us here," Florence says, though her own moist eyes betray her words.

Someone tells me I'll always have a home on the mountain and someone else hopes I find what I'm looking for and I suddenly feel as though I've become the heroine in one of those books I read as a child.

David pours wine and opens beers and smiles at me. He tells me that my open hospitality reminds him of his mother.

"She's a caretaker," he says. "You look after people in the same way."

I think of the time we visited his parents in D.C. and I found his mom sorting through a can of mixed nuts, selecting only the cashews, and putting them in a plastic bag. The sweet, crescent moon shaped nuts are David's favorite, and she wanted to be sure he had enough for the plane ride home. I felt strangely outraged that she would spend so much time on such a silly task. *No way in hell I'm gonna dig through a can of nuts for this guy.* But here I am, making sure he gets an extra dollop of whipped cream on his pie. My urge to look after people is part of the reason I moved home. I wanted to spend time with Dad, but I wanted to look out for La and my brother as well. My decision to move back to Los Angeles is about looking after myself, which is a skill that does not come as easily.

Mountain bedtimes are early even on New Year's Eve, and so most of our guests are gone by ten, leaving David and me and my boys to count down the minutes. We have flashlights at the ready in case there is a black out, but as the clock ticks, we crank up Stevie Wonder and dance together in the kitchen. I twirl into David's arms. He dips me back and plants a kiss on my smiling mouth. No one has to tell me to loosen up because I am loose, my anxiety is at a bare simmer, and it's not just the champagne that's making me feel this way. It's being here in this place that I love and actually loving it again because I will leave it soon.

Still a bit groggy from too much champagne, David and I have gathered on New Year's Day with Mom at Jason and Megan's house for our last dinner in New Mexico.

"I'm so happy for you," Mom says. She loops an arm around David and squeezes him tight.

"I'm happy for me too," I say.

"She's not the only one getting a deal here," David says. "Your daughter is quite the prize."

I resist the urge to sneak out with Megan for a cigarette because I know that David will be able to smell the smoke on my lips. I want to sit on that stoop with her, though, want to huddle together around the lighted match and share a laugh. I worry that we'll lose touch once I move. We don't like to talk on the phone. We don't write enough letters. I know that without our daily contact, we will fall behind on the details of each other's lives.

Jason's fingers are curved perpetually around a red can of Tecate. His eyes are growing hazy. I lean against the bulk of him and he plants a sloppy kiss on the top of my head.

"I love you, you know."

"This is a great night for you and your Dave," he says. "You've got yourself a good guy there. A keeper."

At the end of the night, David helps me into my coat. Everyone has gathered at the front door to say good-bye, but I can't even get the words out of my mouth. Megan looks up at me from beneath a crinkled forehead, her wide, blue eyes shining. She gives me a quick, hard hug. It's the same kind of fierce hug I used to get from Grandma, the kind I get from La.

"You take care of her," she says to David.

I turn to hug Jason, who is suddenly sobbing. He holds onto me, crying into my hair, rocking our bodies together. I hold my brother and tell him it will be all right. Finally, he pulls away and wipes the back of his hand across his face. He takes a deep breath and tells me he loves me and then, still sobbing, he walks out of the room.

"Is he all right?" I ask.

"He'll be okay," my mother says. "You know how he gets."

I do know how he gets. Behind my mother's house is an arroyo (basically a ditch with steep, slanted sides). For most of the year, the earth at the bottom of the arroyo is dry, cracked, and covered with brown pine needles. When we were smaller, the arroyo was a great place to build forts or ride bikes or reenact scenes from Star Wars. After a day of play, we'd return to the house covered with red dust. For most of the year, this was fine. During late summer and early spring, however, we were not allowed to play in the arroyo because an hour of heavy rain could turn it into a raging river, and we could be swept away in the tide. This is how my brother is. His tears come all in a flood, and all the dry months before them make him helpless to absorb the torrent of his emotion.

* * *

The next morning at Tinkertown, the snow is melting in the driveway, and patches of red mud bleed up into the white. I take a deep breath, inhaling the damp smell of snow, mud, and the smoke from the morning wood-stove. The mountain behind the cottage is still dark, waiting for the first rays of the sun to bring color to the piñon trees. My new view will include houses stair-stepped up a steep hill and a line of palm trees standing up like a horse's mane along the neighboring ridge. The lacy boughs of pepper trees will fill in for juniper, and the nostril widening scent of eucalyptus will replace the woody aroma of mulching pine needles and horse manure.

Dad and La join David and me in the driveway.

"Oh, hon," La says. "Travel safe." She hugs me tightly and thanks me over and over again for coming, for being her partner. She is proud of me and happy for me and will miss me like anything. I hug her back and am surprised when I am the first to let go.

Dad and I walk a few steps up the driveway.

"So you're off," he says.

"I'll be back," I say through tears.

"Well, sure you will," he says.

I don't know how much he understands. He is detached, pulling away from me to kneel and give Wallace a good scratching.

When he stands up again, I hug him hard. I press my face into his shoulder and tell him I love him. Though he hasn't said it in a long time, I wait for the response, and when it doesn't come, I whisper it to myself. "I'm mighty fond of you too," I say.

When I pull back he is wiping his eyes.

"I don't know why," he says, "but I'm crying."

Home in Los Angeles * *March 2000*

I HAVE BEEN REPLACED at Tinkertown by a series of caretakers. A woman named Helen makes fresh-squeezed vegetable juice and calls Dad Patrón. In return, he calls her Helen the Melon and foils her attempts to get him out for a walk by accusing her of forcing him on a "death march." Patty comes in the company of her ancient Great Dane and brings paper bags filled with fresh garlic from the fields outside her trailer. A guy named Cal, who lives up the road, takes Dad on fishing trips to the Jemez.

"Fishing? Dad doesn't like to fish," I say to La during one of our weekly phone calls. *Plus,* I think, *Cal always bugged the shit out of Dad.*

"Well, he seems to like Cal," La says.

I am struck by the idea that these people will remember Dad differently than I do. In the last two months, Dad has given up rock runs and taken up fishing. What's next? La tells me he's been nailing bottle caps onto the outside of the cottage. Just as they used to bring bottles to fuel his building need, now all our friends save metal caps.

"It's getting pretty crazy," La says, laughing. "But what can I do? It keeps him busy and happy. He's out there right now."

The distant sounds of hammering come over the wire and I imagine the cottage sparkling in the sunlight, bumpy as a beaded lizard.

La asks if I've found a job and if I've been writing.

"Are you finding your way?" she says.

"I'm trying."

I stop taking Zoloft cold turkey and throw the rest of the sample bottles from Johanna into the trash. But as soon as I stop swallowing the pills, I wonder if I should have had a better plan. As these fragile chemicals fracture and fall away, I swear I can feel my brain vibrating in my head as though suspended in Jell-O.

David is careful with me, coddling me the way he might if I'd just come through a long illness. He tells me I don't have to look for work right away. He tells me to get my bearings. He writes two checks, one for the rest of my student loan and the other for the outstanding balance on my credit card.

"I was lucky enough not to have any student loans," David says. "Besides, this way we can start fresh."

David, it turns out, is a saver. He pays his credit cards off monthly and even has a chunky IRA. It boggles me that he could be so organized.

"It's not really me," he says. "It's my parents. They got me started. I just keep it up." He nuzzles his face into my neck. "I'm your man, baby. Let me take care of things."

I try to take David's advice and relax back into Los Angeles. Every morning, he makes the drive from our apartment in Echo Park across the city to the Santa Monica offices of *Buffy the Vampire Slayer*, where he is a script coordinator. I kiss him good-bye and then curl into my big green chair to finish off the pot of coffee and the paper or head out for a hike up and down the hilly streets of our neighborhood.

One day, I buy a big scrapbook and a packet of photo corners and spend the next couple of mornings sitting at the dining room table reconstructing the last eighteen months. I start with Jason and Megan's wedding where I wore a gray bridesmaid dress and sported a complicated updo. One photo shows Jason carrying Megan over the threshold of their hotel room. He is laughing hard, and Megan's smile could light a dark night. There are pictures of the snowy Aberdeen cemetery where I searched for Grandpa's grave, broom in hand. There is a close up of La and Dad and me that I took just before I moved home. I remember how we squeezed together and how Dad tickled his fingers into my side just before the shutter clicked. On the last page of the album, I paste the photos we took the morning David and I left for Los Angeles.

After I finish the scrapbook, I turn the pages slowly. Already, my time in New Mexico is growing distant. Here in the city, the lights add a purplish glow to the bedroom I share with David, and the sound of traffic fills my ears, crowding out the dark stillness of the mountains.

I call Tinkertown. When I get Dad on the phone, he doesn't realize who I am.

"It's Tanya," I say. In the background, I hear La's bright voice repeating my name and urging him to talk.

"Well, so it is," he says finally. "So it is. Where are you, again?"

"In Los Angeles," I say. I tell him about the warm weather and the books I'm reading. I tell him I've visited the Autry Museum and taken a ride on the ancient funicular downtown known as Angel's Flight. His answers grow shorter and shorter until he is silent.

"Hello?" I say. Over the hum of the long distance line, I hear the sounds of hammering.

"Dad?" I shout. "Hello? Anybody there?" I press my ear to the phone and listen to the sound of penny nails being driven through bottle caps into the wood siding of the cottage. I close my eyes and imagine Dad squinting in the sun, a couple of straight nails held between his lips. He swings the hammer rhythmically. He is doing just what he wants to do. I hang up the phone and hope that eventually I can do the same.

Dad's Walkabout ✻ *June 2000*

"I CAN'T FIND YOUR DAD," La says. I can hear the fear in her voice; can picture her mouth tightening reflexively around the words. "He's gone."

I am naked, pulled out of the shower by the ringing of the phone. I stop breathing for a moment as the word "gone" aligns itself with "missing" instead of "dead." I am dimly aware of David as he wraps a bathrobe around me and leads me carefully to the bed. La tells me that yesterday afternoon Jason dropped Dad off at the fairgrounds where she was competing in a horseshow. My brother didn't take the time to find La; instead, he trusted that Dad could make his own way. But instead of finding La on his own, Dad vanished.

For a moment I have the thought that this all happened because I wasn't there.

Since Dad's diagnosis, Jason has done very little firsthand caretaking, and so he isn't as aware of Dad's limitations. He picks up Dad for lunch or a couple of hours at the tattoo studio, but he has carefully kept himself out of the circle of intense caregiving that La does all the time and I do now on an as-needed basis on my trips home. He doesn't know that Dad has wet himself and that I have taken off his jeans and thrown them into the wash. He doesn't know the agony of watching as Dad peels a bloody scab off a wound on his arm or picks at a small scratch on his nose until it bleeds. He hasn't been around for most of the big fights or for the times when nothing will work and Dad throws things or shouts in frustration.

Before I moved back to Los Angeles, I was angry with my brother for being so detached. Now, though, it is something that I have come to understand. It is nice to be in the world without that constant knot of worry. For me, a couple of states provide the buffer that Jason finds in just over thirty miles. Jason builds ponds in his garden, races go-carts with our cousin, and barbecues on the weekend. He is turning thirty in a couple of months, and he has chosen to put his energy into being in the prime of his life.

"Do you want me to come home?" I ask La.

"I don't know," she says. "I don't know what you can do. I called the police and they're looking. Everyone's looking."

She wants to get off the phone in case someone is trying to call. She tells me she's going back down to the fairgrounds.

I hang up the phone and start to cry. David sits next to me on the bed and holds me tight.

"They'll find him," he says.

"But what if something happens to him?" I ask.

"Your dad is a pretty crusty character," David says. "I mean, I know he's changing a lot, but he's not gonna let something happen to him."

I sit on the sofa with the phone on my lap and wonder if the next time I see Dad, he'll be laid out on a coroner's gurney. A death like this could be considered a kind of accidental suicide. Just after his diagnosis, he told me how he'd like to jump in his truck and blaze off the top of the mountain. "Just check out in style," he said. We talked about the old chief in the movie *Little Big Man* who climbs to the top of the mountain and lays down, saying, "It is a good day to die." Maybe all these early thoughts gathered momentum and pulled him into the path of an oncoming semi. It's possible that his initial urges to "check out" fired up a kind of primitive machinery like the one that drives the aging elephant away from his herd to meet death alone.

I want more time. The doctor gave us five years. I need every day to figure out a way to say good-bye.

Dad has been missing for nearly twenty-two hours when the phone rings again. It's La.

"He's back," she says. She is laughing and crying at the same time. I frantically gesture to David. We hug and cry while I try not to miss any of La's words.

"Something told me to take Old 66 through the canyon," she says.

The two-lane section of Route 66 where La found Dad is about ten miles from the fairgrounds where Dad was last seen.

"I just had a hunch," she says. "And sure enough, about halfway through the canyon, there he was. Tanya, I thought he was a ghost. I thought I conjured him up. He was just walking along by the side of the road."

"He was walking toward home?"

La tells me she pulled over as calmly as she could and even though her heart was beating a thousand miles an hour, she simply said, "Hey, you wanna ride?"

"What did he do?"

"He just kind of waved."

"How is he now?"

"He's sleeping," she says. "He's worn out. And so am I."

"Tan," La continues. "We didn't want to call you. No one wanted you to worry about this. Especially your brother. You should call him. Let him know it's okay."

When I talk to Jason, he is crying.

"Our poppy," Jason says. "What are we going to do about our poppy?"

He tells me that he is so sorry. He tells me that Dad should never, ever be left alone.

"We've got to make a hand-off," Jason says. "You know, from one person to the next. He can't just be left places anymore. He doesn't know where he's going."

I ask Jason not to be too hard on himself. I tell him to get some rest and just give Dad a good squeeze for me the next time he sees him.

"I'm not as good as you, Tanya," Jason says.

"We're all good," I say.

A Short Lead * *June 2000*

A FEW DAYS LATER, I fly home so that I can see with my own eyes that Dad has returned from the missing. I've recently been working a series of temp jobs in L.A. and flying back to New Mexico gives me a sense of specific purpose I find comforting.

La is headed out for a three-day horse show. I can tell by the speed with which she loads her gear into the trailer that it's a much-needed break. While we talk, we both dart glances across the yard at Dad, who sits in a green, plastic lawn chair with Radar on his lap.

"I've kept him on a pretty short lead since his disappearance," La says. "I think I'm driving us both crazy, but I don't want to let him get too far away."

"It's all I can do not to tie a rope around him," I say.

La laughs and gives me a quick hug. She tells me she's stocked the fridge and arranged to have Maggie and Florence on at the museum for extra hours.

"They're on guard too," she says.

After La leaves, I sit in the willow rocker on the front stoop of the cottage and try to mine the facts from Dad's shadowy memory. Though not even a week has passed, he can remember only fragments.

"I was on the back of the motorcycle with your brother. I grabbed onto his belly and held on."

"Where did you sleep?" I ask.

"Oh, just down in the ditch and weeds," he says. "It was dark and good."

I am reminded of the way Radar scratches out a shallow circular bed in the dirt before curling himself into a tight ball of sleep and how the old cat Nick revels in a good dust bath. Dad seems to spend more and more time with the animals. He turns away from our overly verbal ministrations and finds quiet comfort instead in the warmth of Radar's head on his knee or the trusting way Nick offers up his big cat belly.

"I didn't have a car," Dad says. "I didn't need a car. I just walked along, carrying my thoughts."

When I ask if he talked to anyone, he says, "Oh, you know, everyone's a character. But they just think they're characters, they're trying to be characters. They're just walking along, mostly. I just walked along too."

"Did you eat?"

"Sure. I got a beer or two," Dad says. "You know at one of those little holes along in there."

"Where?" I ask. "Which hole?"

"Some people gave me some popcorn," he says.

"What people?"

"This family. They asked if I wanted a ride and they had to drop some stuff off and I said sure and they said hop in. So I did."

"You just got in the car with them?" I say, immediately worrying about what could have happened.

"Sure. Why not?"

When I was a kid, my dad took my hand when we walked. His fingers are thick, his palms wide. His are good hands to hold. When we walked on the road, Dad walked on the outside of me, facing traffic. I remember asking him once why he did this.

"So I can protect you," he said. "If a car comes too close, it'll get me and not you."

At nine, I couldn't imagine living without my father. I hoped that the car would be big enough to take us both.

Dad is picking at the scab over his most recent tattoo. The brightly inked image of Ganesha, the Indian Elephant-Headed God, is ravaged with dried blood. La recently bandaged it, but the raw edges of gauze and tape are too tempting. Once he's peeled them away, his fingernails go to work on the skin, digging, always digging, as if to reach the bone.

His nails are long and several are split and frayed looking. Those on his right hand are crusted with blood.

"It's manicure time." I say this in the same voice I might use to say, "All-you-can-drink beer served by topless barmaids."

"Okay," Dad says as he stands to follow me through the screen door.

The bright voice worked. I feel bad about singing out "time for vitamins," "let's take a pee," "we're gonna ride in the truck," hoping that Dad will behave like a dog cuing his moods off my own. It's worse, though, when my bright tone is met with darkness. Then he'll sneer, "Have you lost your mind?" or tell me to go fuck myself.

I guide him to a chair while I collect a washcloth and a bowl of warm water. In my pocket I have a nail clipper and a handful of Band-Aids.

I sit down opposite Dad and ask him to hold out his hands. He spreads his big fingers wide and lets me run the washcloth over them. La says it's hard to get him to sit still long enough to cut his nails so I know I need to work fast, but he seems to be enjoying the warm water.

"Splish splosh," Dad says. "Warm wash."

I hold his hand in mine and very carefully clip the thumbnail while Dad watches with great interest. He hums quietly while I move on to the next nail and the next.

"We're finished," I say.

"Well, will you look at that," Dad says, wiggling his fingers out in front of him. "Ain't I pretty?"

Though Maggie and Florence spend nearly every day working in the museum gift shop, they still seize upon my visits as an excuse to hang out with Dad over dinner.

"I'm just wondering what's in the oven," Maggie says, as they come into the house. "It smells divine in here."

I've layered salmon over a bed of fennel and sun-dried tomatoes and put together a big salad. Florence sneaks me a bottle of blush wine in a brown paper sack.

"I don't know about you, but after a day in the shop, I could sure use a glass."

I take the wine into the nook that holds the washer and dryer, unscrew the cap, slosh some into a couple of coffee mugs and hand them out to Maggie and Florence. Though Dad is sitting at the table staring right at me, he doesn't seem to register what I've just done. This is new. Despite everything he's forgotten, his ears have always been tuned to the sound of a bottle opening. Not anymore.

After we've eaten the salmon and feasted on cake, we clear the dishes and sit at the table. Florence wants to know when I'm going to get married, and Maggie tells me there's plenty of time. They wonder if I'm doing any writing and whether I'm getting any rest.

"Los Angeles moves pretty quick," Florence says. "That city just makes me tired."

The city makes me tired too. I couldn't get out of New Mexico fast enough, but these visits to take care of Dad are the only time I feel like I'm doing something that matters.

Dad shifts in his seat and looks out the window at the darkening sky.

"We should probably get going," he says. He starts to stand up and looks around as though trying to locate his coat. Florence's eyes widen with concern, but she musters a smile.

"That's a pretty subtle way of telling a couple of chatty old bats to hit the road," she says.

"Dad, you are home," I say.

I can tell he's getting frustrated and so I stand and cross over to him. I take his arm and show him a framed photograph of him with La and his signature on the painting over the big chair in the corner. I lead him into his bedroom and show him his bed. I open the drawer of his dresser.

"These are your things," I say, holding a pair of socks. "These are your clothes. Your books. This is your house."

He looks at me for a minute like I've gone crazy.

"This is all just stuff," he says. "It doesn't mean anything. How can you tell me I live here?" His voice rises to a shout. From the kitchen, I hear the sound of a chair being pushed out across the brick floor.

"You okay in there?" Florence shouts.

"We're okay," I say.

"That's easy for you to say," Dad says. He sits down on the edge of the bed and his shoulders slump. His anger has disappeared and left only resignation. I miss the anger. It ties him to the world and makes me know that some small part of him is still aware of the injustice of his disease. I know what will happen when this anger is gone for good. I've seen the dull eyes and slack face of Grandma Rose and her fellows at Manor Care. When they no longer remember to be angry, they die.

A Very Romantic Table * *September 2000*

DAVID HAS TOLD ME that we will be going to dinner to celebrate my completion of a big freelance writing job, but he hasn't let on where we are going. As soon as we get on the 101, I know he is finally going to propose.

As we head up the twisting road to Yamashiro, the Japanese restaurant that was the site of our first kiss, I try not to smile too much. The valet helps me out of David's old Jetta and I feel like I'm floating. I can't look at David because I don't want this not to be what I think it is.

The hostess winks elaborately and says, "Oh, Mr. Goodman. We have a very romantic table for you. For such a special event." I think that if David could will the floor to open and swallow her, he would. She turns, and we follow the silk bustle of her kimono to a table with a view of the entire city. I am wearing an old navy blue rayon dress that is a little shapeless, but comfortable—the kind of dress you wear when you don't want to jinx things.

We eat beautiful bento boxes of sushi and bowls of pickled cucumber. David holds up the deep fried head of a shrimp.

"You're supposed to eat it in one bite," I say. "Just chomp it."

He takes my advice and stuffs the whole thing in his mouth. He tries to smile as he crunches through shell, antennae, and eyeball. Just as he's mustering the strength to swallow the thing, our server arrives with a bowl of ice cream. A candle glows merrily atop the green mound.

"For the special occasion," she says. "I understand it's a very good night."

We laugh and eat the ice cream. After dinner, we walk out into the terraced gardens. We say goofy things about the view and the dinner and we wonder how long it will take to get our car back. And then suddenly David bobs a little, starts to get down on a knee, then pops back up.

"Almost five years ago on this same spot," he says, "I asked if I could kiss you. Now I have another question."

This moment is awkward and strange and elating. Perfect. David digs around in the front pocket of his trousers and comes up with a ring. It is a single round diamond set in a platinum band. It is exactly the kind of ring I like, which is not such a surprise because given even the slightest opening over the last four years and ten months, I've told him exactly what kind of ring I would like. It had to be simple, almost like a child's drawing of a ring. I didn't want anything artsy and handcrafted. I didn't want a turquoise ring just because I'm from New Mexico. I wanted this symbol to be as real and as recognizable as those school buses lined up outside San Antonito Elementary School. David got that. He got it because he got me.

The next morning, I wake up and make phone calls. I call my dad first. By some miracle he's the one who picks up the phone on the first ring.

"Dad," I say, "David asked me to marry him."

"Well, isn't that something," Dad says.

"It is," I say. "It really is."

"So, here's Carla," he says. I hear a click as he puts the phone down and then the rattle of La picking it back up.

"Hey, hon," she says. "What's the news?"

I tell her. She is excited and happy. We cry a little too, because we don't know what shape Dad will be in for the wedding.

"It's going to have to be in New Mexico," she says. "Your dad can't travel."

La proposed to my dad. He wanted her to leave the house she'd built up north in the tiny town of Cuba, New Mexico, to live with us at Tinkertown. She told him there was no way she was going to do that without a ring on her finger.

"It was a matter of principle," she told me later. "I wasn't coming down there to shack up with your father and take care of you guys. He was the love of my life, but I needed stability."

I understand this. I'm impressed that she could ask for it. She was thirty-two when she married my dad. I will be thirty-two when I marry David.

"It was thanks to John F. Kennedy and the Bay of Pigs that I married your mom," Dad told me one night when I was still living in the Tinkertown house.

"I'm confused," I said.

Dad went on to say that he'd been in the army when Kennedy sent troops to the Bay of Pigs and the men in Dad's unit were told they were going to be shipped out.

"I knew I wouldn't last a day in a real battle," Dad said with a smile. "I was going to be killed and that was a fact."

"So you got married?" I asked.

"Shit, no," Dad said. "But what I did was write the most poetic proposal letter to your mom. I never thought I'd be alive to see it through, but you know that whole thing turned out to be a fiasco. Our orders were canceled and here comes your little mama, jumping off the bus in Colorado Springs with her suitcase packed."

"So you married her?"

"I'm no liar," Dad said. "The best thing to come out of that whole situation was you and your brother. And that's a fact."

I will take David's name, Goodman, and add it to my own. I don't think I can entirely stop being "Tanya Ward," but I want to mark our marriage in some traditional way and I want to share the name of our future children. I test out this new name, writing it over and over the way a teenager might scrawl the name of a boyfriend over the cover of her notebook. My new name, Tanya Ward Goodman, seems to be a sturdy combination of where I come from and where I'm going.

Wedding Dresses and Funeral Parlors
✳ *October 2000*

I MAKE A TRIP to New Mexico. As usual, the descent into Albuquerque is a bumpy one. I look out the window of the plane and try to focus on the blazing yellow cottonwood trees that follow the line of the Rio Grande like a second golden river. In mid-October, the days are still bright with desert sun, but the shadows are longer and the blue of the sky deeper. On the ground, I know that the air will be redolent with the sweet, charred smell of roasting green chile. The wheels of the plane hit the tarmac with a thump and I am home.

"Here comes the bride," Mom sings as I come out through the security gates. She wraps her arm around my waist and gives me a good squeeze. "Let's see that rock." I hold out my left hand and wiggle my ring finger.

Tomorrow there will be a ladies tea at Mom's house to celebrate my engagement. The next day, we'll go look at wedding dresses with Megan. Right now we have to go to Manor Care to check in on Grandma.

"How is she?" Mom asks.

Grandma has been moved from the Alzheimer's wing into hospice care. She hasn't eaten in several days and no efforts are being made to keep her body from slowly shutting itself down.

"Not good," I say.

In an envelope in my pocketbook, I am carrying Grandma's engagement ring and wedding band. Before I moved back to Los Angeles, when Grandma was still up and walking around, she kept taking the rings off. The aides would find them in the bathroom or tucked behind a sofa cushion or at the bottom of a cup of juice. One day, one of the nurses gave them to me.

"Keep them for her," she said. "Or keep them for you. She doesn't even know they're gone."

A couple of weeks later, Grandma looked at her empty finger and said, "Where is it? I had a star there. A little star."

I felt guilty for taking the rings. What did it really matter if she lost them? The diamond, the little star, was just a bit bigger than the tip of a ballpoint pen. La thought we should save them so that Grandma could be buried with them.

"She and your granddad chose to be buried next to each other," La said. "I don't think she'd like to lay down beside him without her rings on."

The curtains are drawn against the afternoon light and the room is dim and cool. I pull a chair up next to the bed and lean over Grandma. Curled on her side, each breath coming shallow and quick as a kitten's, she seems impossibly small. It is as though her flesh has melted away, leaving only fragile bones beneath paper skin. I stroke the tight gray springs of her hair.

"Gran," I say, "It's me, Tanya. I just got off an airplane and came right to see you."

I tell her that I'm going to get married.

"In the spring. You remember David," I say. "You liked him."

I reach out and cup my hands around her curled fingers. She is barely warm and I think I can almost see her life lifting out of her body and disappearing into the air like steam.

I kiss her forehead and her cheek and the stiff cluster of her fingers.

"Travel safe, Gran," I say.

The next morning, while Mom and I are making preparations for our tea party, the phone rings.

"Your grandmother passed," La says. "She's gone."

She wonders if I can meet her at the funeral home with the wedding rings.

"I've got her dress in the truck already. Your dad doesn't really know what's going on. I think he kind of gets it, but I can't really be too sure."

Dad cried really hard when his father died. Though it was almost two decades ago, I remember that day as if not one hour had passed. I was surprised by the intensity of his grief. When he spoke of my grandfather, it was never with love. He told us that my grandfather had been so heartless he left Dad's dog Rusty to die in the street after a car hit him. But when Grandpa died, Dad stayed back in his workshop, alone with his grief. I could hear him sobbing, and the sound of it unnerved me. Up until that day I didn't think that my dad had loved his own father. On that day I started to understand how complicated love can be.

I meet Dad and La at the mortuary. "My ma died," Dad states simply.

"I know," I say. I throw my arms around him, and he stands motionless in my embrace.

The funeral director leads us into a small room and gestures for us to sit in upholstered chairs facing his desk. He asks us about the clothes Grandma will wear, and I slide the envelope containing her rings across the desk.

"You might not want to place anything of value in the coffin," he says softly. "I can't vouch for the care she'll receive in South Dakota."

"It'll be okay," I say. "She should be wearing these."

Grandma will wear the turquoise blue floral dress she bought for my brother's wedding. "It cost nearly fifty dollars," she told me then. "It wasn't on sale or anything." Her hair will be set and curled. Her gold wedding band and the engagement ring with "the little star" will be slipped back on her finger, and she will be put on an airplane and flown back to Aberdeen where she will be laid to rest right next to Grandpa. Like his, her name will be written in pencil on the big paper map of the Aberdeen cemetery.

"Well, that's about it, right?" Dad says.

La reaches across and squeezes his hand. "That's about it, honey," she says.

Dad shrugs and pushes himself out of the chair.

I wonder what he is thinking. He seems to have traveled to a place beyond grief. Dispassionate and remote, he is a spectator now, no longer a participant in his own life. La's eyes shine with unshed tears and I hold her blue gaze for a moment.

La and I decide to fly Grandma's body back to Aberdeen and the trip that started as a celebration of my engagement turns into a journey back to South Dakota for Grandma's funeral. I realize that it is possible to do both. Grandma would appreciate that. She was a thrifty woman and a practical one. She'd be pleased to see that I accomplished so much on one airline ticket.

On the day before La and I leave for South Dakota, I go to look for a wedding dress with Mom and Megan. We've been all over Albuquerque, and we figure we might as well check out Helen's Wedding Belle on Central Avenue. When I was a kid, we'd eat big plates of sour cream enchiladas next door at Baca's Mexican restaurant and afterward, I would look through my own reflection in the big plate glass windows and dream of dancing in those shining white dresses. Today, Helen's seems a little rundown, especially compared to the glamorous wedding shops I visited in Beverly Hills. But I can't afford those dresses.

I try a simple ivory gown with thin shoulder straps and a row of tiny satin buttons up the back. When I come out of the dressing room, Megan jumps out of her chair to hug me. "This is it," she says. She runs down the sidewalk to Route 66 Tattoo Gallery, where my brother works, and brings Jason back to see it.

A few minutes later, my brother's tall frame fills the door of Helen's Wedding Belle. Surrounded by so much fair-colored tulle and lace, Jason stands out like Johnny Cash in a buttercream factory. He wipes his eyes with the back of his hand, and I see that his thumb curves back the same as Dad's. He laughs.

"Well, shit, Tanya, this is really something."

Without taking the dress off, I write out a check for the deposit.

Grandma Returns to Aberdeen * *October 2000*

IT IS PHEASANT-HUNTING SEASON in South Dakota, and all the hotels in and around Aberdeen are booked solid. We arrange to fly into Sioux Falls where we'll stay overnight in a bed and breakfast before making the two-hour drive to Aberdeen the next day for the funeral.

The tiny airport is on high alert for the arrival of the hunters. A banner reads "Welcome Pheasant Hunters," and hastily scrawled cardboard signs point to a "Dog Holding Area" where hunting dogs are treated to bowls of water and kibble inside a ring of bright yellow caution tape.

"It's a bad time to be a pheasant," La says.

Our bed and breakfast is a large Victorian style house on a quiet street. The owners, a fireman and his wife, are happy to see us.

"We don't get much business this time of year. The B&B experience really isn't for hunters," she says as she leads the way up a flight of stairs to a corner room with two twin beds. From the windows, we can see a swing set on the lawn of the house next door.

"I should call and check in," La says. But she doesn't move to grab her phone. The last time we were in South Dakota together, Dad was able to stay by himself at home. This time, we have left him under the watchful eye of La's mom, Connie. Dad calls Connie "Granny Goose" and complains about her smoking. She's a tough old broad with a face as wrinkled as an elbow and a habit of dropping ash from her super slim cigarettes into the upturned cuff of her trousers. She treats Dad like a child, setting up little art projects for him and talking to him in the slow, patient tones of a pre-school teacher. This in turn angers and soothes him. Just before we left, Connie gave me a box of thank-you notes. "Don't forget to write these," she said. "There are going to be lots of reasons to thank people."

While La takes a bath, I lay out my clothes for tomorrow. I've brought a black skirt and white blouse to wear to the funeral. The skirt has a fuchsia pink silk lining. It reminds me of Grandma's neon polyester pants and bright gauzy headscarves.

La returns to the room wrapped in a white towel, her hair dripping wet. "It's so ridiculous," she says, "but shaving my legs in that big bathtub made me cry. I don't remember the last time I did that."

I wrap my arms around La and think of all the relaxing aromatherapy bath products I have guiltily shipped off to her since my return to Los Angeles. I want to apologize for being insensitive. I'm surprised by how much Dad has changed, shocked to realize that he cannot be left alone for even the short span of time it takes to run a razor over your legs. La tells me that she tries to get him into the bathtub, but more often than not, he hops in the hot tub out on the porch and she gives him what he used to call a circus bath with a washcloth before getting him into his clothes.

"I'm not complaining," she says. "I love your dad more than anything. This is what we're doing now . . . It's just nice to have a bath, you know?"

The drive to the funeral in Aberdeen will take a couple of hours and I take the wheel, encouraging La to rest her eyes. Just as soon as we leave the outskirts of Sioux Falls, we begin to see the hunters. In pairs or groups of four or five, they hunch in the fields at the side of the road. They wear tawny-colored camouflage and bright neon orange vests or hats. In the distance we hear the muffled crack of a rifle. "Run, pheasants, run," we shout when we see a startled flock take flight. "Run."

Ten years ago, on a postcard bearing a picture of Wall Drug, one of his favorite roadside attractions, Dad wrote, "It was fun to see this place in November—no tourists, no crowds. We're now in my old home town—no nothing."

In the gray afternoon light, Aberdeen seems drained of color like a black-and-white photo left too long in the sun. We take a drive past Wiley Park where, in high school, my dad used to steam up the windows of his girlfriends' cars and, much later, I played as a child. We drive past Grandma's old apartment and her church and The Flame restaurant, where we had steaks on our last visit. It's closed tonight and looks so desolate that I wonder if it will ever open again. Many of the shops downtown have gone out of business, and those that remain, with their bolts of fabric and flowered china, seem decades out of date. Once Grandma is buried, we won't have a reason to return to this town.

Back home, this place is all Dad talks about. He tells me about building a western town out of cereal boxes with his elementary school friend, Gary, as if it happened yesterday. He weeps for the death of his old dog, Rusty. Tears come to his eyes when he talks about the librarians at the Alexander Mitchell Library. Those women smiled upon his curiosity and appetite for facts. They fed his mind.

Now the library is gone, and so is the Orpheum Theatre, where for twenty cents Dad could see two Tom Mix serials and eat a bag of popcorn. The girls are gone too, the ones with the tight sweaters and soft hair, who parted their lips so willingly in the back seat of a car in Wiley Park. They have all grown up and moved away. As we drive through the streets, I have the distinct feeling that just behind us the road is disappearing, the buildings are folding up, and when we've finished here, there will be nothing on this spot but prairie grass.

Without a coat of snow, the cemetery is smaller than I remember. Brass nameplates are laid down like rivets in the brown grass. It's windy today, and I can hear the ching-ching-ching of the chain hitting the flagpole. A square of bright green Astroturf marks Grandma's grave. Her flower-covered coffin sits on a stand nearby. Three rows of white plastic folding chairs have been set up under a small white tent. So this is it, I think. This is what she saved up for.

On Dad's birthday a year ago, La and I took him to dinner. Just after we sat down, La put her elbows on the table and announced that she had made plans for cremation.

"I contacted the mortuary and got a two for one special, so both your dad and I will be cremated."

"Well, Jesus," Dad said. "Happy birthday, honey."

And again, for the millionth time, I wondered if Dad was really so sick after all.

"I know it's kind of morbid to bring up right now, but I just wanted you to know I've got everything taken care of."

Satisfied that we'd been given notice, she flipped opened her menu and began scanning the options for dinner.

"Well, after that," Dad said, "I could use a drink."

"You and me both," I said.

Grandma's is the first funeral I have ever been to. I've never seen a coffin up close, never thought about what they do with the dirt from such a big hole. As it turns out, they pile it up and throw a sheet of fake grass over it so that you don't think too much about it. The pile looks like a bright green pimple on the surface of the brown grass, and it's about all I can think about. Well, that and the fact that inside that wooden box, my grandmother is wearing her turquoise dress and her shiny gold glasses and, the "little star" of her engagement ring and wedding band.

The relatives begin to arrive, and La and I move to greet them. She whispers names to me as we walk across the grass.

Dad's cousin Dick makes his way slowly across the gravel drive and up onto the grass. He wears a bolo tie with his suit, which reminds me of Dad. Another one of Dad's cousins is decked out like he's stepped off a stagecoach in Deadwood and sports a Wyatt Earp mustache. These men both got little bits of whatever it was that Dad got a whole lot of. This thing compelled Dad to read issues of *Desert Highways* from the 1920s and made it seem like a good idea to trade a week's work for the broken-down carcass of an old chuckwagon. It kept him mixing paint into the wee hours of the morning and kept his fingers moving and moving. I have a pencil drawing that Dad made of an angel in earmuffs flying over a small town. At the bottom of the page he wrote, "The Angel of Raw Talent Makes a Bombing Run over Brown County, Spring 1940." This angel may have dropped the bomb on my dad, but the shrapnel seems to have scattered far and wide in his family.

Dick has a train layout in his basement, but he still works at 3M to pay the bills. The Wild West cousin dresses like a cowboy, but he hands me a card that announces him as a businessman. I wonder if those bits of shrapnel worry at them like they do me. I can feel the need to write under my skin. At times it feels like a surface wound and at others like a gnawing ache deep in my flesh. I want to do it, but I often have to force myself. Dad did not have to force himself. He just picked up a brush or a pencil or a carving knife and the Angel of Talent was there, waiting for him.

The Wedding ✳ *June 2001*

"ARE YOU AWAKE?" La says.

I am awake. I was lying here looking up at the ceiling when I heard her uncharacteristically soft steps on the wood floor outside my room. I am surprised that she is asking. I think of the times when she stormed through my door with such urgency that I wondered if my bed was on fire. I think of David's first visit, when she flew through the door, catching David and me naked in each other's arms. It's a blessing that we weren't having sex.

Today, I am alone. La comes into the room and sits on the edge of the bed. She holds her closed fist toward me and I open my palm to receive her pearl necklace.

"Something borrowed," I say.

We lean together with our arms around each other.

"You're my girl," La says. "You're my girl and you're getting married."

Later there are hair appointments and a bridesmaid's lunch, but I've spent the last hour selling tickets to the museum and handing out quarters for the fortuneteller. It is comforting to ramble around the museum in shorts and a T-shirt eating toast and talking to visiting families. Dad and I sit in twin metal tractor seats under a sign reading "Tinkertown Museum."

"Looks like this is a big thing," Dad says. "Something's really going on."

"I'm getting married," I say.

"Well, how about that," he says. He rests his hand on my knee for a moment. Throughout all our planning, I have been adamant that I want Dad to walk me down the aisle. La is not sure he'll be able to handle it. Mom worries as well. They don't want me to be disappointed. They don't want Dad to be overwhelmed or frightened. I hope he'll rally. The show must go on.

Once, when I was nine, I spent the week with Dad and my uncle Louie at a carnival winter quarters in Coolidge, Arizona, where Dad paid me a dime a hoof for painting the feet of twenty carousel horses. When we had finished the job, we went to Diamond's department store in Phoenix, where Dad and Uncle Louie sat on pink puffed chairs and watched while I tried on dress after dress in the kids' department. We finally settled on a long, Hawaiian-print dress with yellow rick-rack at the neck and turquoise-blue flower shaped buttons down the back. Though I was sunburned and my skin was covered with paint speckles, I saw myself reflected in Dad's eyes and knew I was beautiful. That night, I wore the dress to dinner at the Reata Pass Steakhouse, where we ate big sirloins and iceberg salads with thick blue cheese dressing. When our cowgirl waitress told us that country star Hoyt Axton was seated just a few tables away, Dad winked at me and said, "Well, you tell Hoyt that Miss Tanya Ward is seated over here at this table."

A couple of days ago, I took Dad with me to Helen's Wedding Belle for the final fitting of my wedding dress. Though it was a warm June day, he wore his big, black down-filled coat and a hat stitched with the slogan, "Radar is the Best." He kept his hands in his pockets and hunched his shoulders up around his ears. His hair was long and unkempt and his cheeks were unshaven. When I came out of the dressing room he looked up for a minute, but he didn't stand. He had a kind of half-smile, but I wasn't sure it was directed at me.

"What do you think?" I said. I gave him a spin. In the mirror, I could see my slim waist, the pretty line of my collarbone, and the creaminess of my long neck beneath the short sweep of auburn hair, but I saw none of this in Dad's eyes. He'd gone inward, pushed down deep into himself, tight as a hand in a pocket.

I make the trip from Tinkertown to the hotel where the wedding is to be held crammed into the back seat of my brother's Ford Bronco. Jason and a very pregnant Megan sit in the front, and I share the back seat with my twelve-year-old cousin, Alexandra, and several cases of beer. The drive takes us off the blacktop up a long dirt road. Jason lets out a whoop and steps on the gas, and we rattle and careen over the slippery gravel, our voices vibrating as the tires hit every bump.

The day passes quickly with lunch and flower arranging and the greeting of so many loved ones until I have just a few moments alone after I am dressed. I stand behind a set of tall wooden doors peering out through the crack as the last of my friends and family members settle in their seats. Over the speakers, I hear the sudden drumbeat that opens The Beach Boys' "Wouldn't It Be Nice," and as I hum along, I realize that the wings in my chest, which surely should be vibrating like crazy at a time like this, are completely still.

The plan is for Mom and La to walk down the aisle just before Dad and me, and so we are all waiting by the big door for my music to start. Otis Redding is singing "The Happy Song." I have looped my arm through Dad's when suddenly, Otis stops mid-note and my song, "Searching (for Someone Like You)" comes on. Dad starts to step backward as though he's going to sit down, but before I have time to panic, La grabs Dad's arm and Mom takes my free hand and the three of us propel Dad out the big wooden doors and past the first few rows of white wooden folding chairs. We are all walking each other down the aisle, each of us leaning on the other for support. Dad is in the center, wearing blue jeans, his woven Chimayo vest, and bolo tie. La holds his arm, elegant in a cream silk blouse and long, blue taffeta skirt the color of a robin's egg. Mom laces her fingers through mine. She's wearing a flowing rayon gown in a purple Indian print with chandelier earrings and flowers in her hair. Ahead, I see David standing in the sunshine. I can't stop smiling. *Here comes the bride*, I think, *here comes the bride with her whole big, crazy clan*. When we get to David, La gives me a hug and Mom kisses my cheek. Dad starts to shuffle off, but I grab him and hug him hard and for just a breath, he hugs me back. He is here.

I dance the first dance with my new husband to Paul McCartney's version of "'Til There Was You." I lay my head on his shoulder and breathe in the warmth of him. When he smiles, his eyes crinkle at the corners in a way that I think might make me happy every day for the rest of my life. When the song is over, I start to leave the dance floor. I have read enough wedding magazines by now to know that the second dance is traditionally the father-and-daughter dance. But Dad has grown tired and antsy, and so La has taken him home. David has read these wedding magazines too. He is holding my hand and guiding me to safety.

"Wanna dance?" Jason sweeps me out of David's protective embrace and onto the floor. His dyed platinum hair glistens in the night. He has taken off his suit jacket and wears suspenders and rolled shirtsleeves. His body is loose and fluid in the way that Dad's used to be before the plaques and tangles began to weigh him down. He swings me in and out, twirls me under his arm and laughs as I stumble in my long dress. I have danced with Dad like this dozens of times—a kind of loose jitterbug, turning into a waltz or a two-step. We danced in the kitchen to Dwight Yoakam and Willie Nelson and The Kinks blasting out of the tinny speakers of Jason's boom box. "Let her rip," Dad would say, the smooth, leather soles of his cowboy boots slip sliding on the floor. "Let's kick out the jams." As the song ends, Jason pulls me close and kisses my forehead. He smells like beer and salt and heat. He smells just like Dad.

The Drill * *July 2001*

A MONTH AFTER the wedding, La asks me to stay with Dad for five days while she flies to California to look at retirement communities for her mom. I had already been planning a trip home to attend Megan and Jason's baby shower.

"You can feel free to say no and I won't go," she says on the phone before my arrival. "It's great timing, though. I'd really appreciate it, and I know Mom would. Your dad's been really easy lately. He's pretty mellow."

Her enthusiasm has a familiar brittle quality. I've grown to recognize the sound of her voice when she's had enough.

"It'll be fine," she says. "You know the drill."

The "drill" is basic: feed him, watch him, and keep him from peeing in the front yard or walking on the road by himself. If he brushes his teeth or changes his clothes a few times, so much the better. The drill doesn't change. But Dad does. Every time I visit, he's different. It is impossible for me to prepare for my time alone with him. As impossible as it is for me to say no to La when she asks that I look after Dad. I amp up my own enthusiasm and offer up a grin that I hope La can hear over the line.

"Of course I'll do it," I say. "It'll be great."

"I can't thank you enough," La responds, and if she can't hear my smile, I can certainly hear her relief.

Always a master of scheduling, La has coordinated my arrival to coincide almost exactly with her departure. When I emerge from the Albuquerque Sunport, she and Dad are waiting in the truck with the engine running. I throw my suitcase into the bed of the pickup and squeeze into the cab next to Dad.

"Well, hello there," he says, sounding surprised.

"Hello," I say. "Did you know I was coming?"

"Well, she said something and we got in the truck and here we are," he says.

La jumps out and grabs her suitcase. I slide behind the steering wheel as she comes around the other side of the truck and knocks on Dad's window.

"Hey, Sweetie," she says.

"Hello," he says, then turns to face the windshield.

La knocks on the window again. "Honey," she says, "open the door."

Dad turns to La and knocks on the window from the inside. She laughs and I laugh and our laughing makes Dad laugh. I lean over and open the door.

"You silly guy," she says, snuggling into Dad's arms. "I'll see you in a couple of days, okay? I love you, honey."

"Well, I love you too," Dad says. He seems surprised by his feelings.

La looks up at me, tears in her eyes.

"I've got to go."

She gives Dad one more hug and then turns quickly and walks through the automatic doors into the airport.

"Poof," Dad says.

It takes about forty minutes to drive from the airport to Tinkertown. I fill that time with chitchat.

"I'm a ghost writer," I say. "Hoping to go corporeal soon, though." The joke flies past unnoticed. I wonder if there's been any rain. I talk about the cats. I ask about my brother. Whenever I stop talking, there is silence. He has changed again. Even though it frightens me that Dad doesn't answer my questions, I continue to ask them. "What shall we have for dinner?" I say. There is a pause. "I was thinking we'd barbecue something. How's that sound?" Dad is silent. He pulls his seatbelt out away from him and holds it so that it no longer touches his body. Finally, I ask, "How's Radar?"

"Best dog in the world," Dad says. He lets go of the seatbelt and lapses back into silence.

As a kid, I lived for time alone with my dad. "Wanna take a ride?" Dad would ask, and minutes later we'd be whizzing down the road. He'd hold his hand out the window, cupping the air. He told me it was like feeling the breasts of angels. We'd drive to the hardware store on the corner or all the way into town. It didn't matter how far we went, it just mattered that we were sharing the narrow space of the truck's cab. When we were together, nothing bad could happen.

I look across at Dad. His graying hair is oily looking and tangles at the back of his head. His beard and mustache are trimmed, but his cheeks and neck are only haphazardly shaved. The buttons of his long-sleeved, pale blue shirt strain over his belly. On his feet are dirty, brown boots with unevenly threaded and elaborately knotted laces. His cheeks are slack and his eyelids motionless. Even in sleep there is evidence of the encroaching emptiness.

As I pull into the driveway of the house, a few raindrops spatter the windshield. Dad stirs and then wakes with a start when I cut the engine.

"We're here," I say brightly.

"What the hell do you mean?" he asks.

"We're home."

Radar rushes out to the truck, springing up to greet me as I open the door. "Look," I say, "here's Radar."

"Well, Radar," Dad says. He pats the seat of the truck, and Radar hops in and licks Dad on the cheek. Dad laughs.

"Let's get in the house before the rain comes," I say.

"Fuck no," he says. He goes back to petting Radar.

I take a deep breath and come around to Dad's side of the truck and open the door. "Hey, Dad, are you hungry? You want to come inside?"

Dad looks at me and looks at my purse. "You want me to put my dick in that?" he asks.

I try to laugh. All the books say that the caretaker should remain positive because the Alzheimer's patient reacts to the caregiver's emotions. For this reason, La and I have made a point to stay upbeat even when times get tough. If we laugh, sooner or later Dad laughs, and it's okay again. At least this is how it worked the last time.

"Well?" Dad says. He's not laughing.

"I'd just like to go inside," I say. "It's starting to rain."

"So go," he says. "Get the hell out of here." His eyes are narrow and his lips curl maliciously. I find his face ugly and this makes me want to cry. I turn and take a few steps away from the truck. When I turn back, Dad is out of the truck and looking up at the sky.

"It's raining," he says. His voice is gentle now, and his face is smooth and placid.

"Yep," I say. "We should go inside."

"Should," he says. The clouds let loose and I grab Dad's hand and pull him the last few yards to the house.

Inside, I towel my hair and then, Dad's. When I remove the towel, he automatically takes a small, black comb from his back pocket and smoothes his hair off his forehead to one side. It is a gesture I have seen hundreds of times, one so familiar it is possible to be hardly aware of it, but this time, I am supremely aware. How many more times will he perform this simple act of grooming?

"What are you looking at?" he asks, scowling.

"Nothing," I say. "Are you hungry?"

I open the refrigerator and rummage around. It is too rainy and I am too tired for barbecuing. I dig out a block of cheese and some bread and tomatoes.

"Grilled cheese sound good?"

"Gooder booder," Dad says and laughs.

"Terrific," I say. I grate cheese and heat a cast-iron skillet. I slather the bread with butter and slice tomatoes and begin to feel myself relax. I should have expected a rough patch at the beginning. It must be confusing for Dad to have me arrive and La leave. I'd be angry if someone showed up and put David on an airplane with no explanation. After we eat, things will settle down. We just have to get back into a routine. While the sandwiches brown, I fill glasses with water and slice some melon. Dad watches me silently as I slide a sandwich off the spatula onto a plate and put it in front of him.

"Get the hell out of here," he says.

I try to smile as I sit down next to him with my sandwich. Dad glares at me as I take a bite and chew slowly. I ignore him, and he looks away from me, out the window. A few moments later, he looks down at the sandwich in front of him and says, "What's this?"

We sit and eat in silence. I watch as Dad uses the edge of his fork to cut his watermelon. I count the extra seconds it takes him to spear the melon and lift it to his mouth. He is concentrating. His lips move cautiously around the food. Radar sits next to Dad's chair, his eyes fixed on my father. He has all the focus that Dad lacks. The dog reaches out a tentative paw and places it on my father's leg. Dad turns, surprised to see Radar.

"Well, hello there," he says. "Hi little guy. Are you hungry?"

He offers Radar a bit of watermelon, but Radar turns away. I stand and grab a box of dog biscuits from the counter, shaking out a pile on the table in front of Dad.

"Try these," I say.

Dad picks up the biscuit and hands it to Radar, who takes it gladly.

"There's a good dog," Dad says. "Best dog in the world." He smiles, not exactly at me, but for now it is enough. I don't need to ask any more questions. I just need to sit here quietly and savor the peace. Outside, the storm clouds are blowing over the mountain, leaving behind a night scented with damp earth and green grass.

I try to be patient. I do. But it's hard. I want more from Dad than is reasonable to expect. I feel angry that he is leaving and I feel angry that I am being left. I pour this angry energy into sweeping the kitchen. The brick floor is uneven and dips in the center, making it virtually impossible to keep clean.

"There's mud here," I say. Mud and dust and dog hair. In New Mexico, the earth is the color of salmon flesh and when mixed with a summer rain creates deep red stains on anything it touches. I want to go back to the city where the dirt is covered with cement and grass. I want to go back to the smooth wood floor of my apartment and to the clean white sheets I share with my husband.

At the back of the refrigerator, I find a couple of regular beers and a nonalcoholic beer—a Sharp's. Because Dad has forgotten what the refrigerator is for, we don't have to hide the beer any more. At one time it would have made everything much, much easier, but tonight it saddens me.

"Hey, Dad," I say. "Feel like a beer?"

Nothing. And then as my words sink in, he turns toward me.

"Well, isn't that nice," he says. "Wouldn't be half bad."

I open the Sharp's and set it down in front of him, then turn to pour my own beer into a glass. Dad takes a sip and then turns the bottle in his hand, inspecting the label. I wonder if he'll notice that it's a Sharp's, the brew he once derided as "weak as tea and twice as nasty."

"Good stuff," he says.

"Yep." I raise my glass and clink it against the lip of his bottle. I'm feeling bad that I'm this desperate to share something with him.

After a few sips, he puts the bottle down on the table and folds his hands again. I'm surprised. It has been a long time since I have seen Dad stop drinking a beer. Generally when drinking anything—water, milk, juice, but especially beer—he swigs it down in one long, continuous swallow.

"Are you finished?" I ask.

"Am I what?"

"Never mind." I need to stop asking questions. I need to sit still and just be with Dad as much as he will let me. I sip my beer and look around. Dad's artwork is hung almost floor to ceiling on every wall. The painting he did for La when they married of two eagles in flight, their talons locked together, their wings forming a heart, hangs next to a painting of Radar dressed as the pope, surrounded by raccoon choir boys. The pieces he did at the onset of his illness, including a self-portrait called "No Longer Mine," incorporate the images of his SPECT scan. In the scan, the brain is divided into sixteen brightly colored slices. When he was first diagnosed, Dad found faces in these sections and called them the sixteen little brothers. In his self-portrait, he stands at the dark mouth of a mine out of which emerge these ghostly faces, hovering in the air like so many tribal masks.

Dad shifts in his chair and stands. He heads swiftly through the living room and out the back door. I follow. He stumbles ahead of me and stops just around the side of the house where he unzips his jeans and pees on a rock planter. I turn away, wanting to give him some privacy, but also needing to know exactly where he is. He's been peeing outside since we got home from the airport. It's nearly dark now, so when he comes back in the house, I turn on the bathroom light and leave the door wide open.

"Here's the john," I say.

"So?" he asks.

"In case you have to pee. It's getting too dark to go outside. Besides," I say, affecting the Old West voice we joke in, "it'll be a darn sight more civilized than peein' in the woods."

"Pee-pee-pee," Dad says, laughing.

I laugh then too.

Dad laughs harder and starts to walk toward me, holding his hands out in front of him like Frankenstein's monster. He rolls his eyes and growls. He grabs me then and starts tickling me hard. I laugh and tell him to stop, but he won't. He keeps tickling me harder and harder. It's starting to hurt.

"Hey," I say, "quit it."

"Quit it, quit it," he says, holding on to me harder.

"Dad." I twist out of his hands and move away from him, but he chases me, pushing me into a corner and grabbing my belly, my sides, and digging his fingers into my armpits. I'm feeling scared now. He's so much bigger than I am and, in this strange, blank haze, so much stronger.

"Hey," I yell. "Back off."

"Fuck you," he says. "Fuck you."

My eyes burn with salty tears. "I'm sorry," I say. "Let's just relax, huh? Let's just simmer down."

The screen door bangs. It's Nick, the cat, pawing at the door to be let in.

"Well, Nicky, you big old cat," Dad says.

He scoops up the battle-scarred tabby and sits down at the table. Nick purrs as Dad turns him gently onto his back and rubs his belly.

"There's a good fellow," Dad says. And just like that, the scary robot Dad is gone.

At nine-fifteen, I decide it's time we turn in. I head to the bathroom and put toothpaste on both Dad's toothbrush and my own.

"Here you go," I say. "Come on in here and we'll brush our teeth."

I am surprised when Dad stands, takes the toothbrush, and follows me easily into the bathroom. I turn the water on and begin to brush my teeth. In the mirror, I catch a glimpse of myself exaggerating my brushing motion like some kind of freak. I've got to tone down this preschool teacher bit. Dad sort of chews on his toothbrush and then holds it under the running water.

"The last fine on the dusk of eeny splak," he says.

"What?"

"What what?" he says.

"Okay, great," I say. "Let's get to bed."

I take his hand and lead him into his bedroom. I switch on the light and pull back the covers. He sits down on the edge of the bed and lets me take his shoes off.

"You want to take your jeans off?" I ask.

He just stares at me, so I stand him up and unbuckle his belt. In an attempt to make this less awkward, I narrate the whole thing, but he doesn't seem to care. He stands quietly while I unbutton his jeans and slide them down. He holds on to my shoulders and steps first one leg out and then the other. I try not to look at his bright red briefs. Instead, I focus on the eyes that Jason tattooed on the tops of his feet. I take a deep breath. We're almost in bed, I think. One day down, four to go.

"Snuggle in here, Dad," I say, pulling back the sheets. He slides his legs under the covers, but sits bolt upright, looking at me. He's still wearing his blue cowboy shirt.

"Do you want to take your shirt off?" I ask, reaching for the buttons. He slaps my hand away.

"Okay, but can I take some of this stuff out of the pockets?" As Dad looks down with interest, I reach into his pocket and come up with two small sticks, a pen, a wad of paper towel, a Band-Aid, a photo of La, a folded postcard of an "art car," a square plastic bread-bag clasp, a small ball of tissue containing two screws, a rock, a penny, and, strangely enough, my reading glasses.

"Wow," I say. "That's a lot of stuff."

"A lot of stuff. Stuff, stuff, stuff. All this is just stuff," Dad says.

I put everything in a row on the top of the dresser and turn back to Dad.

"Do you want to lay down?"

I rearrange the pillow for him a bit and try to help him slide down so that his head will be in line with the rest of his body, but the best we can do is a sort of neck-breaking slouch. Suddenly, I'm obsessed with getting him to lay down flat. I want him to notice that he's not comfortable. I want him to understand that this is a crazy position for sleep. I want him to protect himself even if just from a stiff neck.

"Hey, there," I say, "Can you just scrunch down?" I tug at his shoulder and motion down toward the bottom of the bed, but he just looks at me and shakes his head.

"Nuh-uh," he says.

"Okay, then," I say. "I'm turning off the light." I reach up and switch off the lamp above his head. It's a clamp-on spotlight attached to a plywood cutout of my dad. He painted himself naked and reaching for the sun. On the opposite side of the bed, another spotlight is held by a painted version of La. She's naked too, her blonde hair in a jaunty bob, her hands stretching up to the sky. Looking at Dad's bent shape, I envy La her intimacy with him. If I were his wife instead of his daughter, I could climb into this bed and drag him down into the sheets in my arms. I could make him rest by holding him next to me. As Dad's speech disappears, all that is left is touch, and there is a limit to how I can touch him. I lean close and kiss his forehead.

"Good night, Dad," I say. "Sleep tight." He doesn't respond.

I climb into the fold out bed in the room next to Dad's. I try to read, but realize after going over the same sentence a dozen times that I am too tired. I switch off the light and stare out the window at a star-filled black sky. In a moment, I'm asleep.

I don't know what time it is when I hear what sounds like a hard rain. Radar is barking and the cats are meowing. I don't want them to wake Dad, so I jump out of bed and rush out into the living room to quiet them. It's still dark, but in the light from the bathroom, I can see Dad in the middle of the living room. It's not the rain, I'm hearing. It's Dad peeing like a racehorse on the brick floor. Radar is jumping around him, still barking, and I don't know what to do. So I wait. I wait for a long time while Dad pees and pees. When he finally stops, Dad stays where he is. He seems almost to be sleepwalking. I slowly approach him.

"Dad," I say quietly. "Let's get you cleaned up, huh?"

I take his hand and lead him into the bathroom where I run warm water in the sink and grab a washcloth. He hadn't taken off his underwear so they're soaked through and his legs and feet are wet. I give him a quick scrubbing and then try to take his underwear off, but he pushes my hands away. I give up. I wrap a towel around his waist and lead him back to his bed. He's asleep before I've turned the light off.

Back in the living room, I go at the floor with hot water and bleach and a mass of paper towels. Radar wanders around me with questioning eyes.

"It's okay, buddy," I say. "Just a little accident. Go on back to bed."

He heads into Dad's room, where I can hear him jump up on the bed and spend a few moments scratching the blankets into a comfortable nest. Before I go back to my own room, I stand in the doorway of Dad's room and listen to his even breathing. He's asleep, and curled next to him, like a bright spot of moonlight, Radar sleeps too.

It's 12:45 when I climb back into my rickety sleeper-sofa. At 2:03, Dad's up again. I get out of bed and watch as he makes it across the living room to the bathroom and then back to his room. He makes this same trip at 3:15, 3:56, 4:35, and 5:10. At 5:40, Soccer, the old skinny cat with the failing kidneys, begins to howl. I get up and find her clawing at the box of cat food in the kitchen. I open a can of food and set it down in front of her, put on water for tea, and then sit at the table and wait for it to get light. I just don't have the willpower to try to go back to sleep.

When Dad wakes up, he's still wearing his red briefs. I decide the best thing to do is to get him into the bath. As I begin to fill the tub, the sound of running water draws him into the bathroom. He leans against the edge of the sink and watches the water.

"Looks pretty good, huh?" I say.

I turn off the water and leave him alone in the bathroom. Outside, I perch on the arm of the sofa and listen for sounds. I hear the cupboards open and close and the toilet flush and then a few quiet splashes. I wait a few seconds and then peer around the door. Dad's sitting in the tub with his legs straight out in front of him. He's paddling his hands through the water on either side of his body. The back of his hair looks oily and knotted. "Hey, there," I say. "Can I wash your hair?"

He sits still with his back straight while I carefully rub shampoo into his scalp. He's been using tubes of bright green Prell shampoo for my whole life, together with Right Guard deodorant, Crest toothpaste, and Listerine mouthwash. These and wood shavings, WD-40, turpentine, enamel paint, and beer are the smells of my father.

"Lean back a little," I say. "I don't want the soap to get in your eyes." Dad remains straight-backed and stiff, so I hold a towel over his face and try to rinse the soap out of his hair. When I'm finished I put a clean towel on the edge of the tub.

"Take your time," I say. "Here's a towel for when you get out. I'll make some breakfast."

He's quiet this morning so I try to be quiet, too. I talk too much; always trying to fill in what I think is empty space. Yesterday, Dad looked right at me while I was in the middle of some extended ramble and said, "Martha." Martha is Dad's aunt. According to him she could "talk the hind leg off a deaf mule." Today, I'll try to take the hint.

When La finally calls to check in, her voice has none of the forced bravado she had used to assure me that Dad was "real easy."

"It's terrible here," I say. "He's changed so much."

La lets out a choked sob. "I know," she says. "I know. But it's the kind of thing I thought you should see for yourself."

"Thanks for the heads up," I say. I am feeling ambushed. I want to shout, "Jesus, Carla, what the fuck are you up to anyway?" but I don't. Instead, I listen and nod.

"I got to Mom's and fell asleep for twelve hours. I am wiped out," La says.

"And I know why," I say. "I'm not sure he should be at home anymore. I don't think it's safe. For him or for us. It's too hard."

The phone line goes silent for a while, filled only with little sniffles.

"I think you're right. I thought you would see that," La says.

She tells me there is something called a respite program at the nursing home where Grandma lived. She thinks it might be a good test. I wonder if she was worried that I would be angry with her for wanting Dad to go to Manor Care. Maybe to feel okay about her decision, she needed me to be on board. After only a few days, I am convinced. I don't know how she does this every day, all day by herself. I am amazed by her bravery and grateful to her for doing her best to keep Dad safe and in his own home, but now "home" has no meaning for Dad. It's time to move on.

On the morning of my third day in New Mexico, Jason calls to tell me he's stopped drinking. He says he's made it through three days without a beer and he's feeling clear enough to declare that he's not drinking anymore.

"It's been ten years since I've made it through even a day, you know?"

My brother is thirty years old. Although I am aware of his ability to make short work of a case of Tecate, I had no idea he'd been drinking so much for so long.

"I don't want to have to drive Megan to the hospital with ten beers in me."

"I'm proud of you," I say. "It'll be great to experience things as your real self."

"I don't know if it's my real self," he says. "It certainly isn't what I'd call the norm."

His voice is quiet and serious, so different from his usual bluster. He sounds scared. He tells me he has a headache.

"You need to drink water," I tell him. "Lots of water."

"I don't like water," he says. "I don't honestly know what to drink now."

"We'll figure it out," I say and hurry off the phone.

On the way to the baby shower, Dad and I stop at the grocery store and I fill a cart with nonalcoholic beverages. I buy bottles for their funny labels or for the bright color of their contents. I think of my newly sober brother as though he were an alien landing on a new planet and try to imagine what would look most friendly.

When we arrive at my brother and Megan's house, I feel as though I, too, am landing on a new planet. The past three days up in the mountains have been so quiet that the surge of chatter hits my parched soul like a cloudburst. Megan is wearing an orange linen dress, the fabric stretched taut across her round belly. She is like a little sun.

"We brought lots of beverages," I say. "To celebrate."

"This is some wacky stuff," Jason says holding up a bottle of bright pink liquid. "Are you trying to send me back to beer?"

I spend the party following Dad from room to room. I make him a plate of pasta salad and barbecued chicken and sit near him with a napkin and a glass of lemonade. I lead him to the bathroom and keep him from emptying the contents of the medicine cabinet into the sink. I steer him away from the big cooler of beer on the back porch and watch him so that he does not slip out the front gate whenever a new guest arrives. I have brief, interrupted conversations with my friends and family. I cannot exactly share this day with Dad, but because I am with him, I cannot share it with anyone else.

The last streaks of pink drain from the Sandia Mountains as the sky deepens from turquoise to indigo. My brother wanders around the yard, igniting tiki torches with a long butane lighter. Megan has slipped out of her party sandals and scuffs around the porch in fuzzy slippers, gathering together the last bits of pastel-colored wrapping paper and ribbon. The party has ended. The baby is coming soon.

"In all the fuss, I forgot to show you this," Megan says. She hands me a square of thin, slick paper. "Looks like she's ready."

It is a printout from Megan's last ultrasound. The baby's nose is pressed against the inside of Megan's womb the way she'll press her nose against the glass of car windows and pastry cases. Her eyes are open and her wide mouth seems to be curved in a smile.

"You've really got a baby in there, don't you?" I say. "She's so beautiful."

I look across at Dad, who has settled into a chair. He is still for a moment, staring out across the yard at the flickering of the lamps. Jason crosses toward the beer cooler and then turns and heads in the opposite direction and takes the chair next to Dad. We sit quietly, and I try to focus on this moment, really soak it up. We are all travelers here, borne by time and change to new places. I imagine that the baby shifts in Megan's belly, straining her eyes, as we do, for a glimpse of the future.

Breathing Room * *September 2001*

I HAVE A NEW NIECE. The baby's name is Hedy Rose and she is just under a month old. In the short time that Hedy has spent growing accustomed to the arid climate of her new home, Dad's two-week trial run at Manor Care has become permanent.

I wasn't here when Megan began her first contractions, wasn't here to witness my brother emerge from the delivery room, his face flushed with love in the first moment of fatherhood. I wasn't here when La and Jason packed Dad and his suitcase into the truck and drove away from the museum. It's strange to return to such a familiar place and find so much has changed.

"That first day, Jason and I didn't know if he got it," La says. David and I have just stepped off the airplane and now the three of us are squeezed along the bench seat of the big diesel truck headed toward the nursing home.

"But then, just before we left, he sat down on his bed and flipped us the bird with both hands." She laughs, but her voice catches in her throat. "Oh, he got it all right. 'You guys put me in a nursing home,' he was saying, 'Well, fuck you.'"

Ten minutes later, we leave our suitcases in the truck and snap a leash on Radar to walk across the parking lot. La and David stand beside me as I punch in the combination to the Alzheimer's unit. I think of all the mornings Dad and I opened the museum together, Dad shouting the combination to the lock before I could get to it. He wanted me to know he was still there, still with it.

Inside, David holds my hand as we walk through the hallways looking for Dad. Radar runs ahead, his collar jingling, his tail up at full alert.

Though it's been almost a year since I visited Gran here, very little has changed. There's still a crib filled with stuffed animals and baby dolls in the hallway just outside the dining room and a couple of hampers overflowing with white sheets near the nurse's station. The smell is familiar too. It is not unlike the smell in a middle-school cafeteria—a top note of bread and meat covering a base note of cleaning fluid.

"You won't believe it," La whispers, holding tight to my arm, "but he fits right in."

A few minutes later, when we find Dad asleep in the common room, I see that she is right. Though he is at least fifteen years younger than the other residents, there is no discernible difference. He is wearing sweat pants and slippers and his hair is mussed in the back from sleep. One of the aides is leading the gathering through a game of hangman on a dry erase board.

"Presidents," she shouts, her marker squeaking out lines across the white surface. "Seven letters."

Everyone shouts out different letters. Someone says "two." Someone else says "Montana." In the corner, a white-haired woman rocks a small teddy bear and sings in a low voice.

The aide fills in a couple of "Ls" and the letter "I" and then says, "Rail splitting. Stovepipe hat. Beard. Freed the slaves . . ."

"Lincoln," says a tall man with a booming voice. "Abraham Lincoln."

The aide congratulates him and then writes in "Lincoln." "Okay," she says, "How about the first president?" She draws more blank lines.

"Anyone got a letter?" she asks.

The tall man with the deep voice shouts, "Lincoln. The answer is Lincoln."

I let go of David's hand, cross to Dad, kneel next to him, and touch his knee.

"Hey, Dad," I say. "It's me, Tanya."

He opens his eyes.

"Well, so it is," he says.

I'm not sure whether he recognizes me or is agreeing with me. Throughout my life Dad has had lots of names for me. I was The Kid, and Punk. I was Scallop O'Hara to his Rat Butler. I was Holly to his Brad when we reenacted scenes from *The Greatest Show on Earth*. I was Princess and TW and Tanya, Queen of the Jungle. I would settle for any one of these names right now, just for the chance to be pinned into his world, but instead I take his smile and hold on to that.

"You wanna take a walk?" I help him up out of his chair, and we shuffle past the other residents to where David and La wait in the door.

I think back to the day that Megan and I spent driving all over Albuquerque looking at Alzheimer's facilities for Grandma. When we found Manor Care, we thought we'd found a perfect place for Gran to wind down her days. We could not imagine putting Dad here.

"Your dad doesn't belong in a nursing home," La said then, and I agreed. We thought he was different. In the end, though, Alzheimer's is a great equalizer. At Manor Care, Dad lives with mathematicians, businessmen, and farmers. A woman named Elizabeth speaks only German, but it doesn't matter because her roommate can barely remember to speak English. They share custody of a blue teddy bear and murmur to it in gibberish. At Manor Care, bankers trade their suits and well-shined shoes for pajama pants and slippers, mothers no longer remember to care for their children and college professors wear adult diapers and immerse themselves in the simple act of folding and re-folding a towel. Now, Dad is one of them, his eyes cloudy, names and dates slippery as minnows in his mind.

The four of us walk slowly together, letting Dad set our pace. David holds my hand tightly, casting me sideways looks, trying to gauge my reaction. I am waiting to see how I feel about this. Maybe it is because I have already walked these halls with Gran or because I've seen for myself the way that Dad no longer fits in at Tinkertown, but this is not as hard as I expected.

After a few trips up and down the hall, we wind up in Dad's room. He settles onto the edge of his narrow twin bed and Radar immediately jumps up on his lap. We talk about the increased security at the airport and our bumpy Albuquerque landing. We talk about baby Hedy and the end of the season at Tinkertown. Dad watches us talk and then suddenly stretches out in his bed. A second later, he begins to snore. La stands, rearranges his pillow, and straightens out his legs so he looks more comfortable. It is time to say good-bye.

In the truck on the way back up to Tinkertown, La's nervousness reveals itself in a stream of nonstop chatter she keeps up all the way through the canyon and up North 14. When we pull into the driveway, I understand why she might be nervous. It was easy to fit the latest version of Dad into the generic setting of Manor Care, but it is much harder to subtract him from Tinkertown. His body may be absent, but his creative mind is in evidence on every inch of this property. Now, I feel the tears come. I hold David's hand tightly as we follow La up the front walk of the cottage.

"I've been clearing out," she says, almost offering an apology for her neatly made bed and the absence of Dad's collages and pile of scrapbooks. The kitchen table is bare save a large, blue decorative platter, and the windowsill behind it no longer carries its load of pebbles, shells, and rusty screws. "I don't want to put everything away," she says. "But I feel like I need a bit of breathing room so I can get a handle on this."

I unload our bags of groceries and start water to boil potatoes. David moves quickly to help. He digs around in the utensil drawer for a paring knife and begins to peel. He is as comfortable in this kitchen as he is in our own.

"You okay?" he asks.

"Yep," I say. I look out across the yard to where the plum trees are hung with bright blue bottles and watch Radar prance across the dry grass, stopping by habit to lift his leg on the rock where Dad carefully lettered the words, "pee rock." Inside, around the windows, the walls are paneled with old barn wood that Dad salvaged. As much as La has tried to clear out the cottage, Dad remains.

David and I and La sit at the table in the backyard of the cottage and laugh. We open a second bottle of Pinot Noir. Just as I wasn't sure what my reaction would be to seeing Dad at Manor Care, I wasn't sure how this night would go either. Now, we've eaten mashed potatoes and spinach salad and steaks off the grill. The wine is loosening our tense muscles and setting our laughter free into the dark night.

La tells us that just after she married Dad, she sat on the bench seat of the old blue pickup while he opened the mail. When he came to a Visa bill, he wrote "deceased" on the envelope and threw it out the window.

"I remember being so shocked," La says. "I'd never seen such utter disregard for rules. It was thrilling. But at the same time, I thought, *holy shit, this family needs me.*"

I'm thankful to La for paying bills and making sure I applied to college. I'm grateful to her for knowing that if Dad was going to realize his long time desire to run a museum, he was going to need a partner to keep the books. Throughout their marriage, she provided a kind of scaffolding to support his work. She let him focus on the things he was good at and took care of all the mundane details. Now she fills out forms for medical aide and arranges for doctors' visits. She researches new drugs and keeps Dad supplied with clean socks and underwear. Manor Care is an extension of the framework La has created for Dad. It is one where he is safe and comfortable and where he can continue to live as freely as his disease will allow.

The next day, David and I visit my brother and Megan and Hedy Rose. My niece has soft, pink lips that purse into a tiny "o" as if offering a kiss to the universe. Her head is so small, it is easy to imagine she has no memories at all. Right now, only the scent of milk and the warmth of friendly arms smudge broad strokes across her new mind. I wonder if Dad's brain will rewind back this far, if, as he folds into himself, he will find comfort in the primitive sense memories of an embrace, a full tummy, a good stretch.

David holds Hedy carefully, so aware of her weak neck and her inability to support her noggin. I watch him shift her expertly into the crook of his arm and suddenly my own need for a baby makes my face flush.

Megan laughs. "You've got the baby bug." She punches my arm.

"Do not," I say.

"Don't lie to us, sister," Jason says. "You better watch out, big Dave. She's a time bomb looking to explode."

"Okay, so I want a baby. It'll happen. There's time."

"You'd be a good mama," Megan says.

Hedy starts to cry, and Megan takes her from David's arms and holds her close. Jason leans over them, singing in a soft voice.

Hedy gets her middle name from Grandma.

"I wanted Rose to have another shot at a fun life," Megan says.

I think we're all getting another shot at a fun life.

On the plane ride home, David and I use each other as pillows and close our eyes. The way he falls immediately into sleep is something I alternately love and find incredibly annoying. While sometimes, his tumble into unconsciousness abandons me to the swirl of worries in my head, today I am happy to feel his breathing deepen. It is not that he is without worry, it's more that he feels capable of dealing with whatever comes. Though I have always been a worrier, I am starting to understand that I might be capable too.

When I was nine or ten, my parents had one of their huge parties. Our house overflowed with women in patchwork skirts, men with beards, the clink of bottle against glass, the sweet smoky scent of marijuana. Early on a band set up in the corner of the living room, but as the party wore on my parents loaded the stereo with a stack of records ready to drop into "Jumpin' Jack Flash" or the long wailing riffs of Jimi Hendrix. I carefully threaded my way through a room loud with laughter and conversation and crowded with heated bodies. When I got to the stereo, I gently lifted the needle from the record and moved the stack of LPs to one side. When I set the needle back down, Simon and Garfunkel started to sing "Parsley, Sage, Rosemary and Thyme." The room grew quiet for a moment, and then I heard my dad laugh.

"We're getting a little rowdy for the kid," he said.

He crossed to me, cupped his hand around the back of my neck and smiled down.

"You hanging in there?" he asked.

I nodded and leaned against him.

Later, when I got older, Dad would tell me to "loosen up." Once when I poured the last of his beers into the sink, he said I was turning into a killjoy just like my mother. My brother, too, would tell me to lighten up. In high school he'd come home from dates with hickeys blooming like rosebuds on his body. I envied these hickeys, but disapproved of them too. My dad joked that he must be dating a vacuum cleaner.

The summer before I went to college, I took a job as a camp counselor. I developed a crush on a dark-haired, guitar-playing, Birkenstock-wearing senior counselor who told me I needed to "loosen up." For him, this "loosening" included a trip into the woods, after all the campers were asleep, to drink some beers with a handful of other counselors. I agonized over joining them because beer drinking was against the rules, and I didn't think it was responsible to leave my campers with only a younger counselor to watch over them. But ultimately I went. I drank half a can of warm Budweiser and watched my cute counselor make out with another girl before going back to my sleeping bag with a bad taste in my mouth. In the morning, we were all fired.

My default setting is not "loose." I realize that now. It makes sense that I would come home and look after Dad just as it makes sense that Jason would spend hours tattooing him, but not know he can't be left by himself. The best service we can do for each other is to realize that we each bring something different to this experience. When La told me she didn't have time to be compassionate, she was being truthful. It was all she could do to keep the museum running and feed the dogs and the horses and look after Dad. "We're doing all we can do" was our mantra when I was living at home. We all adopted it and said it over and over and over to reassure ourselves and to help us forgive each other. It is only now, though, that I am starting to understand that doing all you can do, even if it doesn't seem like very much, is enough.

Good Company * *February 2002*

I'M STANDING IN FRONT of a huge shelf of pregnancy tests and feeling as nervous and embarrassed as I did buying condoms in college. I've been dizzy on and off for days, but this morning I couldn't even shift in my chair without the feeling that my light head would drift clear away from my neck. Since we've been "trying" for only two months, it doesn't seem possible that I'm pregnant, and so I decide to buy the most inexpensive test, figuring I shouldn't waste cash on the first of what may be many trips to the pharmacy.

Back at the apartment, I walk quickly up the stairs with the test shoved deep into my purse. I don't want to stop and talk to our neighbors. I don't want anyone to know what I'm up to. I just want to pee on this stick, realize I'm coming down with some kind of bug, and get it over with.

Five minutes later, I stare at the bright pink plus sign in the window and try to come to grips with the fact that sometimes you get just what you want right off the bat. I call David at work.

"Lovey," I say. "I'm pregnant."

"What? Oh, wow," he says. "Holy shit. That's great."

"Really? You really think it's great?"

"This is what we wanted, right?"

We laugh nervously, and I wish I'd waited to tell him in person so I could see his eyes.

For most of my life, the idea of having kids seemed pleasant, but nonessential. From time to time, I indulged in little fantasies—me and the baby staring blissfully at the camera or pushing a stroller down the street, the baby's chubby arms and legs reaching for the sun like flowers in a bouquet. No poop, no late nights, no pain in evidence. Quite truthfully,

I didn't know if I could handle all the heavy lifting. Now, after helping to look after Dad, I am pretty sure I can. How could an eight-pound baby have any tricks up his sleeve that I haven't already seen coming from my old man?

After we got married, I told David that I wanted to have children right away. I was already seven years older than my mother was when I was born. I was about to lose my dad. I wanted to get my own kids out into the world so I'd have as much time to spend with them as possible.

At our first appointment, the doctor shows me a tiny twitching blip on the screen. Roughly the size of my pinky fingernail, our child already has a beating heart. I don't know why I am so certain, but I know he is a boy. I feel suddenly as though my world has righted and things are back to the way they are supposed to be. After spending so much time caring for Dad, it will be a great relief to care for our child. It will be a great solace to hear his first word and an even greater one to see him collect new words every day after.

Such a Good, Good Man * *July 2002*

"HE HAS A BIT OF an erection," La says.

"It's okay," I respond, and I mean it. This is not the worst thing. We had arrived at the nursing home to find Dad smelling of shit and perspiration.

"He doesn't want to get changed," the nurses said. "We tried to get him in the shower, but he's having a hard day."

"We can do it," La said. We grabbed some clean clothes out of his closet and then each took one of Dad's hands and led him into the shower room. "Splish splosh," he said, watching with a kind of detached amusement while we took off his sweat pants and T-shirt and unfastened his diaper. La led him into a shower stall, leaving me standing on the damp black rubber flooring.

"How you doing?" La shouts over the running water.

"I'm good," I say. I pick up the diaper and roll it into a ball and drop it into the trash. I am six-months pregnant and my belly has taken on the roundness of a full moon, finally filling out the maternity clothes I've been proudly wearing for months.

From the shower, La keeps up a constant stream of conversation. She can't wait for me to see the flowers she's planted at the museum. And our water tank herb garden has really taken off. She says she's not sure what we're going to have for dinner.

What we're not talking about is tonight's dinner guest.

A couple of weeks ago, La called to tell me she was thinking of going on a date with a man who was not my father. She asked if I thought it would be all right and then burst into tears. Through my own tears, I told her that of course it would be all right and I couldn't be happier for her.

"I like to be part of a team," she said. "You know that your father is the love of my life, but I don't want to be alone. I'm a partnership person. That's just how I work best."

Eric is a planner. He works for a big company that is turning the small mountain community where I grew up into a suburb of Albuquerque. He's the guy who makes sure that the big new houses going up out past my old elementary school in San Pedro Creek are situated in such a way as to insure privacy for the wealthy occupants, who want to take best advantage of the amazing views. He helps make sure that the water needed to fill the swimming pool and irrigate the golf course doesn't lower the already sinking local water table. La opposed the development. When she went to a meeting to register her protest, this tall, soft-spoken fellow from Phoenix caught her attention.

Dad shuffles across the wet floor. La tries to wrap a towel around his waist, but he swats her hands away. Sure enough, he's got a pretty big erection, and his hair is wet and standing on end from being toweled off. "We need to get you dressed, honey," she says and then turns to me. "I'm a little embarrassed."

"Don't be," I say. "Thank heavens something still works."

La laughs. "With your dad, it's not such a surprise."

We maneuver Dad onto a dry area and manage to get a clean diaper on and then support him while he pulls on new pants and a T-shirt. "You look sharp," I say. He turns at the sound of my voice. In the last months, he has stopped holding his head up. His chin rests almost on his chest, rounding his shoulders and forcing him to look up and to the side when he wants to focus on anything. In recent photos, La is often in back of him with her hand under his chin, holding his face up to the camera.

We emerge from the shower room and start our slow progression down the tiled hall to check on the construction project next door. From the window at the end of the hall, you can see the humped form of the Sandia Mountains, which today are a deep purple against a turquoise sky. A few wispy clouds leave white smudges just above the highest peak. This is what would have grabbed Dad's attention last year, but today it is the roar of a front loader at the construction lot next door. He knocks on the window and then lets his hand drop.

"Looks like the building is really coming along," La says. "I only hope it doesn't block too much of the view."

Dad turns away from the window and places a hand on my belly. I look up in surprise. He flattens his palm against my shirt and then traces a circle over my stomach. I stand very still. His hands are smooth and pale, his wide fingernails clean and pink. I have never seen his skin so clean or so soft. Without the almost constant barrage of paint thinner, cement, and sunshine, his hands have returned to an almost childlike softness. These are hands that do not work. As he moves them over my belly, this is the first time I think he might have a vague understanding of my pregnancy. "That's your grandson," I say. Dad says nothing, but continues to caress my belly. Then, just as quickly as he started, he turns and walks away.

"Do you think he gets it?" I ask La.

"I think he does," she says. "But he doesn't know exactly what to do with it. Things have stopped connecting in a way that makes sense to you and me, but I think he's still taking things in."

I look down at my belly and then at Dad as he walks away from us.

"Your dad would have been a great grandfather," La says. "You just have to know that he's going to be there somehow."

"I know," I say. And then we're both crying and hugging. And just as quickly, we're laughing sheepishly and wiping away our tears. After five years of crying, it seems we've gotten this emotional release business down to a science. Dad would have been impressed by the efficiency of his "weeping women."

Dad wanders into his room. He sits on the edge of his bed, his head bowed down, his shoulders rounded.

"Hey, aren't these great pants?" La says. She sits down next to Dad and smoothes the fabric of his elastic-waist pajamas. They're black with orange and red flames running up both legs.

"Real hot-rod pants," La says. "Target. I couldn't resist. Your dad would have loved them."

And there it is again. The past tense. Does he love them now? Truthfully, I don't know. While Dad appreciated the work of artists like Ed "Big Daddy" Roth, the fast and loose, rock 'n' roll hot-rod style seemed several decades ahead of where he felt most comfortable. He preferred the mud-spattered glamour of the circus tent and the low-tech violence of the Old West. I understand why La bought them, though. They are not your standard navy track pants, and La has chosen them to give the rest of the world a cue. Ross Ward would not have stood for the bland beige walls and serviceable blond furniture in this room. He liked to add things to generic motel art. He'd paint in a flying saucer above a desert landscape, a family of skunks parading across a print of Monet's Giverny garden and once a cloud of bats flying out of an old barn that escaped the frame and smudged the walls of the hotel room. "It was a boring painting," he said. "And then it wasn't."

Dad stretches out on the bed, and La readjusts so that she can sit next to him and stroke his hair. He closes his eyes. The skin covering his eyelids is stretched and thin, puckering like a deflated balloon. Though some of his fellow residents are old enough to be his parents, he will be gone long before they are. Because I've been coming to Manor Care for nearly two years, I recognize the signs. I know this silence, this gray pallor. His lips are losing their pink, his green eyes sinking in and growing cloudy. In a process the Alzheimer's literature calls "shrimping," his body is curving in on itself. He is, with marked speed, returning to a fetal state. And when he gets there, when his body is curled tight against the world and his eyes no longer see, he will die.

I am sitting in a rocker, my hands folded over my round belly. It is comfortable to rest this way. My palms seem drawn to the warmth and life that is growing inside me. On the bulletin board next to me are a few photos of my niece, Hedy, and a birthday card I sent to Dad on which I drew in crayon a flaming birthday cake. The drawing is cheerful, but childlike. I can draw a little, but I did not inherit what we have always called Dad's magic hand.

La looks up at me. She blinks back tears.

"When he looks like this, I can't help but think that this is what he'll look like when . . ."

"I was thinking the same thing," I say.

"It's hard not to," she says. "I've been telling him I'll be okay when he goes. I want him to know that."

When she says this, I suddenly feel a rush of relief. I have been thinking this, but have been unable to say it aloud. My father's death was once unthinkable, the kind of thing that would pull me gasping from sleep, a drop into dense, unknowable darkness. Now, I am starting to make out shapes in that darkness as pinpricks of light start to force their way through.

I pull myself out of the chair and sit next to La and lean my head against her shoulder. Together we look down at my father, focusing on the slight breath that makes his chest rise and fall.

"This is a good man," La says.

I was in third grade when I lost my best friend Jennie to a fire. It was just before Christmas. A space heater shorted out and set her house aflame. Jennie's mother and her boyfriend escaped, but nine-year-old Jennie, with the straight, dirty-blond hair and a nose full of freckles, was trapped in her room. She was the first person I ever knew who died. I remember crying into the shoulder of my dad's blue denim shirt. When I'd cried myself out, he presented me with a small box wrapped in a red cotton bandana.

"It was going to be for Christmas," he said, "but I thought you could use it now." I untied the bandana and opened the box. Inside was a silver ring shaped like a crouching frog.

"Here, let me," Dad said. He took the ring out of the box and slid it onto the ring finger of my left hand with the frog's face pointed toward my right. "That way he can watch you draw," Dad said. "His name is Fear-Not. He's a protector. He's gonna make sure nothing bad happens to you."

"Fear-Not," I said.

"That's right," Dad said. "And if he stops working, you've still got your old dad."

I didn't take the ring off until just after I graduated from college. After over a decade of constant wear, the narrow silver band wore thin and finally split. Underneath, my finger was indented. When habit moved my thumb to twirl the ring, I found only an empty spot and the smooth flesh of my finger. I kept the broken ring in a small box, which was lost when I was robbed in San Francisco. Despite the fact that the thieves took nearly everything I owned, it was the loss of Fear-Not I felt most acutely.

I look down at my left hand. On my ring finger, fitting comfortably into the spot once occupied by Fear-Not, is my wedding band.

"I'm looking forward to meeting Eric," I say.

La smiles. "I'm excited too," she says. "You don't think this is too weird?"

It is strange to think of La sipping margaritas with Eric while Dad drifts through the hallways of Manor Care, but I'm not sure the right people appear in your life at the most convenient times.

Back up at the cabin, I sort through the refrigerator and try to come up with some sort of combination that will lend a festive air to this evening. I line up a carton of eggs, two zucchinis, an onion, a triangle of Romano, and a bag of salad greens. Of course there is bread. La always manages to have a good loaf of bread and plenty of butter.

"I'm thinking frittata," I say.

"Great, great," La says. "I'm sure whatever you make will be fantastic."

She wears a sheer white blouse I sent for her birthday a month ago. I bought it just after she told me about Eric. We hear the deep rumble of a pickup truck coming down the driveway.

"He's got a diesel, too?" I say.

"I know," she says. "It's too cute, huh?" She heads out the door, almost running down the sidewalk to greet Eric as he gets out of his truck. From just inside the screen door, I watch her give him a quick kiss before grabbing his arm and steering him toward the house. She is nervous. And so am I. I think that Eric, as he walks into my father's house on the arm of my father's wife to meet my father's daughter, must be the most nervous of all.

Eric is not my father. He is tall and thin with such fair skin and light hair that he seems almost transparent. He wears a pale blue oxford shirt with a button-down collar, khaki slacks, and slip-on loafers. He's the kind of guy my dad would have branded as one of the "shirt-and-tie crowd" when he was feeling nice and as "a dick from the city" when he wasn't. Eric reaches out to shake my hand and I pull him into a hug instead.

"Welcome," I say. I am big and round and warm and full of love for this man who is returning the sparkle to La's eyes.

I am waiting for the cast-iron skillet to get really hot. That is the secret to making a frittata. It takes patience and a slow flame for the eggs not to stick. Through the big picture window, I can see them at the picnic table under the plum trees. They are laughing, their heads bent together over their joined hands. Above them, dangling like crystalline fruit, are dozens of empty glass bottles that Dad wired into the trees. The rocks he gathered on our many "rock runs" have settled into the ground where he left them, the two stone lines coming together to form a closed end. Grass grows up around them. Just as I move the eggs from the stovetop into the oven to finish, the screen door bangs against the frame and then bangs again and Radar bounds into the kitchen. He stands on his hind legs and paws my skirt.

"Hey there, good dog," I say. "How's the best dog in the world?"

He looks at me with his dark eyes, and I rub the silk of his ears between my thumb and forefinger. I cannot touch this dog without thinking of my father's hands, without letting my own hands making the same caressing gestures. I hold the dog's small face between my palms.

"And what do you think of all this, buddy? Who knew, right?"

I don't even know what we talk about. I am too nervous, too determined to put Eric at ease. I do know, though, that while we sit at the metal picnic table with the Sandias growing darker and darker behind us and the windows of the cottage starting to cast glowing squares of light across the yard, I become more and more aware of La's loveliness. It is like watching a fire start. Her eyes soften and her mouth curves more easily into a smile. She is hesitantly flirtatious, taking care to gauge both Eric's response and her own. A little rusty at this game of love, she seems to tremble on the edge of her powers.

From the fold-out bed in the guest bedroom I can hear the roar of Eric's pickup as it wheels out of the driveway. La comes flying back into the house and collapses like a giddy teen on the end of the mattress.

"So, what did you think?" she asks. Her cheeks are red, her mouth swollen from kissing. She was out in the driveway for a long time.

"He's great. Plus, so into you."

"You think?"

"Oh my God, yes," I say. "He just stares and stares . . ."

"He does, doesn't he?"

She grips my arm in her fingers and I squeeze her back.

"We talk," she says. "I realize how quiet it's been around here. Even before we moved your dad, I'd just sit at the table and read while we ate. Now I just talk and talk. Sometimes he stops me. He says I don't have to get it all in today . . ."

"He's right," I say.

"This is a good thing, right?" she asks. She is suddenly teary.

Just after Dad and La were married, we were headed to the hardware store in his old brown truck. I reached over and pulled a long, blonde hair from the sleeve of his navy sweater.

"Hey, wait a minute," he said. "Gimme that." He took the hair and smoothed it back against his arm. "That's one of my lady's hairs. Leave that be."

"This is a good thing," I say. "Dad loves you. He wants you to be happy."

The next morning, we are at the back door of Manor Care. We find Dad asleep in the common room. He is wearing gray sweat pants and scuffed leather slippers. His hands are folded neatly in his lap. La kneels next to his chair and strokes his arm.

"Hey, hon," she says.

He opens his eyes. "Well, aren't you pretty," he says.

She hugs him tightly, rubbing his back for a minute before helping him to his feet.

"Let's take a little walk, huh?"

Dad shrugs. I take his other hand and the three of us shuffle out of the common room and down the hall. We pass Elvira who is a great whistler and Mr. Dorrell and Janelle who are always holding hands. Elizabeth, with the snowy white hair and pink cheeks, sings a song in German about elephants. Dad doesn't seem to notice any of these people. He's humming under his breath. His head is bent, his eyes cast down.

Still holding hands, we stop at the window and look out on the construction site and the mountains beyond. It is a quiet moment. We're all out of things to say. I can feel the baby shift and roll. The movement travels across my belly, creating a little ridge that rises and falls like a whale surfacing. Already I have a sense of who this child will be. He jolts and twists, arms and legs flying out in all directions. There was one whole day when his foot stomped with drumbeat precision on what felt like the inside of my cervix. It was a strange and intimate feeling, electric and invasive. His head is often lodged up under my ribcage. I imagine him there, his ear pressed against me, the sound of my heartbeat like galloping horses all around him.

Dad rubs my hand with his thumb and then looks up. For a moment, his green eyes look right into mine and I think I see a spark of recognition.

"Hey, Dad. Hello," I say.

He holds up first one hand and then the other, noticing that he is still linked with both La and me. He carefully wriggles out of our grasp and then takes our hands and interlaces them together. When he is satisfied that La and I are well connected, he gives our joined hands a little pat. His head sinks forward and his eyes grow vague as he turns from us and begins the journey back down the hall.

Roscoe * *November 6, 2002*

I CRAVE MACARONI and cheese. Not the gourmet goat-cheddar macaroni so popular in the Los Angeles comfort food movement, but the gooey, crayon-orange macaroni my great-grandmother used to make. My belly feels like it is resting on my knees as I waddle through the grocery store asking where they keep the bright yellow boxes of Velveeta, finding it finally on a dusty shelf. Cheese so processed does not need refrigeration.

At home, while I wait for David to make the long commute, I cut the cheese into blocks, marveling at its slight springy quality—like a rubber lizard or a hi-bounce ball from a vending machine. I mix the cubes with elbow pasta, add a couple pats of butter, pour milk over it, and bake it until the top is brown and crisp.

For years this was my birthday dinner. My brother would ask for Chateaubriand and Crab Louis, but I always wanted macaroni and cheese and frozen peas. Tonight, I eat two heaping bowls and drink glass after glass of cold milk. It is the most delicious meal in memory. Yes, I have spent thirty dollars on four separate kinds of cheese to make my own super fabulous version of this down-home treat, but never before tonight, in the company of my husband and my pregnant belly, has anything tasted as good as this South Dakota specialty.

After dinner, David and I sit on the sofa. My belly is so huge, I can only fasten the top three buttons of my pajama shirt. I fold the fabric up over the taut roundness. It is incredible to feel the heat radiate through my skin. Under my palm is the rounded lump that is an elbow or knee. Right now, our boy is curled up inside me. His eyes are open and he is awash in the waters of my body. When I close my eyes, I can see him. I can't wait to meet him, can't wait to hold him in my arms and inspect all his tiny parts. I want to open his gently clenched fingers and massage the soft spot at the base of his neck. I want to put his toes in my mouth. I want to read him stories and give him his first spoonful of ice cream. I want to crash through piles of leaves with him and show him how to stand very still and look closely for lizards sleeping in the sunshine. Like my father did for me, I will make up songs for my boy and help him curl his fingers around a pencil.

The phone rings. It is La. Her voice is bright and brittle and I know that something is wrong.

"Your dad's had a stroke," she says. "He's not in great shape. I don't want you to worry, but I want you to know."

Dad doesn't know that Theo is about to arrive. He is floating in his own waters. Though we find this brine vast and uncharted, I have to believe that he is taking as much comfort and nourishment from it as my son is taking from the fluids of my womb.

Our baby is not due for three weeks, but perhaps because he knows something I do not, he decides to arrive early. At ten o'clock the next morning, I stand up from my chair and feel a small pop. My pants are wet, and for a moment, I think, *great, not only am I huge, I'm incontinent too.* Then I realize the water keeps coming. Holy smokes, this is it. I'm oddly calm. I change clothes and call my doctor's office. Then I call David at work.

"Honey," I say. "My water broke. I'm fine. We have a doctor's appointment in an hour."

"I'm leaving right now," he says. David doesn't sound quite as calm as I feel. In the background, I hear a cheer. This is his first job as a writer on a television show, and I know that he's sitting around a big conference table with the other writers trying to come up with stories that will take three super heroes through another day.

While I wait for David to arrive home, I pack a few things I think I might need for labor. All the books have giant lists of things like lollipops and ChapStick and tennis balls to roll on and music to push by, but now that it's actually happening, all I can think of is my toothbrush. My son's head is acting like a cork, keeping the amniotic fluid from escaping in a tidal wave. As I walk around, he bobs a bit, releasing a drizzle here, a dribble there. I am having small contractions, but they are not painful. My belly feels taut like the string on a bow just before the arrow is let fly.

"First babies never come fast," my doctor says. It's a little after two o'clock and I'm sitting on an absorbent pad with a white paper sheet over my lap.

He holds up a strip of paper that the acidity of the amniotic fluid turns blue before our eyes.

"Your membranes definitely broke," he says. "But you've got lots of time. Go home. Rest. Relax. We'll see you in the morning."

Though we have had nine months to prepare for this event, we are not ready. We have a crib and clothes and a menagerie of pale pastel stuffed animals, but we do not have a car seat. If we do not have a car seat, we cannot bring our child home from the hospital. We pour all of our nervous energy into the pursuit of the perfect seat.

"Let's go to Babies'R'Us," I say. "I could use a walk."

"Let's look at *Consumer Reports*," David says.

"I don't mind browsing," I say. I take a deep breath. The contractions are starting to hurt more. They are also starting to be closer together.

"I think we should figure this out," David says. He's online, checking various websites and shouting out specifics while I walk through the apartment gathering things for my hospital bag. I pack two impossibly small shirts with snaps at the crotch and a tiny flannel blanket and a hat with a pea pod embroidered on the front. I'm aware that I am breathing harder and that the pains are sharper.

"Honey," I say. "I don't think I want to walk around anywhere after all."

And this is how we send our bachelor neighbor off to Right Start to buy the most expensive, highest-rated car seat and how I curl into a ball on my yoga mat and try to breathe through my contractions.

I call my mom. "I'm in labor," I say. "The baby is coming."

"What should I do?" she asks.

"Get on a plane," I say. "We'll see you soon."

I call La. "The baby is coming," I say.

"Holy shit," she says. "It's good timing. Hang in there."

I call Megan. "The baby is coming," I say.

"And you're talking on the phone?" she says. "Geez, Tanya. Just keep breathing."

And I do. A couple of hours later, I make the journey down the steps from our apartment to the car on the street. I have to stop every couple of breaths to bend and let the pain crash over me. Big changes are afoot. I am an earthquake. Our boy is on his way and there is nothing I can do but give myself over to the rumbling.

We will name our child Theodore Roscoe Goodman. Theodore for the nature-loving president whose enormous biography has been weighing down David's bedside these long nine months, and Roscoe for my dad. Roscoe is the name Dad created from his given name, Ross. It is the name he scrawled across the bottom of some of his brightest and happiest paintings and the name that bears little trace of his cold Aberdeen childhood.

At the hospital, I walk around and make jokes, and every few minutes, I curl up into myself and let Theo try to work his way out. It is painful and difficult, but we are in it together and I love him already for his courage and his ferocity. As the contractions come faster and faster, I close my eyes between tremors and I see my son swimming toward me. I rest in these moments. I reach out to my boy and guide him through the water. When I awake, I push with all my might.

Our son is coming. Like a fish, his body is flying quick and silvery through one world into the next. The pain of this transition is almost unbearable.

"Feel his head," my husband says, guiding my fingers down between my legs to something damp and wrinkled and fuzzy like a peach.

"You should see your face," David says. "You look wonderful."

And then Theo is in the world. He is wailing and I am gasping and all around me the lights are dancing with halos made by my tears. We have a son. We have a family.

I bring our boy home in the middle of a rainstorm. From where I sit in a wheelchair in the ambulance bay of the hospital waiting for David to bring the car around, the world looks like a damp and dangerous place. Dingy smog-tinged runoff spills through the downspouts and drips off the open door. Puddles iridescent with oil shimmer across the asphalt. A homeless man wearing a large overcoat and a layer of trash bags secured with duct tape shuffles by the door, ducking his head against the rain. A woman with a wracking cough is pushed by on a gurney. The warm, flannel bundle on my lap seems far too small and too light to hold the life of a human being. I curve around Theo, tucking him against my belly and brushing my lips against his forehead. He looks up at me with sea-colored eyes. I feel like we've known each other for years.

The first few days of Theo's life pass liquidly as we shuffle around in pajamas and slippers, watching the rain bead against the windows of the apartment. We cook big casseroles and kick up the heat so we can unwrap our little bundle and examine his body. He stretches out on the bed, spreading his toes like a cat. Sometimes he wails so loudly that his face turns deep red. We call him The Angry Beet and hold him against us, cooing songs of nothingness and love into his shell-like ears.

"Your dad is dying," La says. "If you want to see him, you should come home."

I am holding the phone in one hand and my son in the other. I rock slowly from side to side like a boat bobbing along on the surface of calm water. Like a metronome set to ticking, my body automatically starts this movement as soon as Theo is in my arms.

"He's in hospice," she says. "It may not be long."

When I get off the phone, I grab a sheet of paper towel to blow my nose.

"I thought they weren't going to tell you," my mother says.

"I think they have to tell me," I say. "I don't see why they wouldn't."

"We didn't want you to be worried."

"I just want to see Dad," I say. "I want him to meet Theo."

At our first visit to the pediatrician, we ask when six-day-old Theo can travel.

"My father is dying," I say. "I need to go home."

Our pediatrician is prone to corny jokes and silly voices. He has a toy koala bear clamped to his stethoscope and sports the darkly slick hair of a 1940s gangster. Today he is perfectly serious.

"Go see your dad," he says.

We prepare to fly home at the end of the week.

That night I sit up in bed nursing Theo. My milk has come in with a vengeance and my breasts are huge and stand out from my body like water balloons, even when I am flat on my back. Theo makes squeaky sucking sounds as he nurses. One arm is tucked against me and the other drifts up, his tight fist bouncing against my chest. I am so amazed by our child. His head is warm and soft and pulsing softly with so much life. I suddenly start to cry and I can't stop. I hear David's quick footsteps coming from the living room.

"What's wrong, lovey?" he asks.

"He's just so beautiful," I say. "I want to keep him safe."

"Of course you do," David says. "And he will be. He is."

"I just don't want him ever to be sad," I say.

"I don't think there's anything you can do about that," David says.

"I miss Dad," I say.

David makes his arms a circle around our new son and me and holds us both until I can't cry anymore.

It is still dark when the phone rings. I know who it is and why she is calling. David is on the phone for less than a minute before hanging up and spooning his body up against my back.

"Lovey," he says. "That was La. Your dad died."

I keep perfectly still. For my whole life I have had nightmares about hearing this piece of news. Where once I could let these night visions evaporate in the morning sunshine, they have been slowly gaining weight and now here they are, fully realized in the wan gray light of the seventh morning of my son's life. I start to sob. David holds me and lets me drench his shirt with my tears. Beside me in the bassinet, Theo begins to stir. He is ready for his first breakfast.

A few minutes later, I am sniffling and red-eyed and sitting up in bed with pillows propped at my elbows feeding my sweet son. Mom shuffles into the bedroom from her makeshift bed on the living-room couch.

"Dad died," I say.

Her face crumples into sorrow, and she sinks to the edge of the bed. With my free arm, the one that I am not using to support Theo, I hold her close and let her cry.

Getting Home ✳ *November 13, 2002*

WE ARRIVE AT THE AIRPORT with a note from Theo's doctor that says it is okay for him to travel. He wears a warm hat, two pairs of socks, and is wrapped tightly in a flannel blanket decorated with cowboys on horseback. As I walk across the shiny, white tile floor, I swear I can see germs coming at us like a blizzard in the headlights. Every few feet someone asks how old the baby is and when I tell them they register shock and surprise. "Awfully young to travel, isn't he?"

"My dad died," I say. "I'm going home for the funeral." Some seem careful not to intrude further on our sorrow while others take a quick step back as if such a strange and tragic situation might be contagious.

I hold tight to my son and watch David bustle ahead to check in our luggage. A black-and-white horse on a karabiner is clipped to his belt loop and when he walks, the toy bobs rhythmically. He clipped the thing on as we were leaving the house, following the advice of some friends to have toys available on the plane. Seeing him do this gave me the same comfort as seeing him with a dishtowel over his shoulder in the kitchen. Today marks the one-week anniversary of his being a dad.

On the airplane, we settle in with Mom at the window and David on the aisle and me and Theo in the middle.

"I just hope his ears are going to be all right," Mom says. "Now you remember, you've got to nurse when we take off." Her eyebrows knit together and she leans in to tuck the blanket more firmly around her grandson.

"I remember," I say. "It's not a long flight."

"Well, it will be for him if he's in pain," she says.

I can feel my left breast start to leak. Milk is soaking through the nursing pad and making a dark circle on the front of my olive-colored blouse. I can feel blood seeping into the pad between my legs. Theo snuggles against me, turning his face toward the scent of milk. I undo my shirt and bra and slip the soggy breast pad into an airplane barf bag.

"That's it," Mom says. "Eat, little guy, eat."

But Theo just toys with my nipple, letting it bob in and out of his lips. Each time he lets go, milk shoots out in all directions. In the last few days I have learned that the human nipple is built not like a plastic baby bottle with only one hole, but instead like a watering can.

"Hey," David says, "you got me."

The engines begin to roar and Mom shifts in her seat, leaning in further.

"Come on, Theo, eat, eat," she says. "Oh, God," she says as we pick up speed on the runway. "Oh, God, his ears, his ears," she says as we feel the wheels lift off the ground. "Is he in pain?" she says as we climb higher and higher into the sky. "It must be just excruciating."

Theo is asleep. He sleeps through the entire flight. He is not in pain. He is content. Just like my dad, he is already a traveler.

We've Got You Covered * *November 2002*

IT IS DARK when we pull into the driveway at Tinkertown, but the lights on the boardwalk are blazing, and the museum doors are wide open. A drifting plume of wood smoke smudges the deep black of the evening sky above the cabin. Megan comes down the front walk to greet us and though her wide, clear forehead is creased with sorrow and worry, her eyes are bright when they land on the wee head of our son.

La hustles out of the museum and up the driveway, still moving quickly through this day and into the night. She pulls me into an embrace and then reaches for Theo. I pass him to her, wanting her to lay hands on him, to take some comfort from this small, warm body. Jason throws an arm around my shoulder and looks down at me, his eyes shiny with tears.

We move into the cottage as if one organism, everyone reaching a hand to touch, or leaning a shoulder, all hungry for contact, for comfort. Inside, our good friend Chris makes me a plate of tuna salad and crackers. Studded with cranberries and lightly dressed, the tuna is the most delicious thing I have eaten in days.

"Theodore Roscoe," Chris says, flipping her waist-length braid over her shoulder. "That's some moniker for such a tiny fella." She leans over my son and touches his head softly with long, tapered fingers.

"You know your grandpa was a good friend of mine," she says to Theo. "I was with him in Australia when he came up with Roscoe." She tells us that she and Dad and La were wearing hooded yellow slickers against an intense rainstorm.

"There we were running around like a bunch of looney birds in this rain and no one could see and Carla kept looking for Ross and shouting 'Where'd Ross go?' and your grandpa, that old kook, kept dodging behind her and saying 'Roscoe? Where's Roscoe?'" She looks up at us through her tears and shrugs her delicate shoulders. "It seemed pretty funny at the time."

The house is warm and brightly lit. Candles burn on the mantel and scent the air. The kitchen counters overflow with baked goods and boxes of chocolate. Flower arrangements bloom on the table, all evidence that our small mountain community has reached out with a bounty of love and condolence.

Chris makes sure I am fed. La makes sure I have a glass of water at my elbow whenever I sit down to nurse. I eat the tuna salad. We are all working to connect ourselves to one small detail, one small task so that we will have some tether, no matter how flimsy, keeping us attached to the world. These everyday details are what keep us moored in times of stress and sorrow. Like David seeking the perfect car seat before the birth of our son, these things give our brain something to do when our hearts are working overtime.

David and I are sleeping in the cottage with Theo. We are sleeping in the bed that Dad shared with La. She is sleeping across the street in a rented house with Eric. Though it is strange to share the grief of my father's death with this man, I cannot help but be impressed by his careful regard for our family. He has made himself a kind of invisible comfort, bringing wood for the fire, washing up the supper dishes, and helping to proof the obituary that La and I wrote together. His respect for our entire family was in evidence when he double-checked to be sure we had included my mother in the printed list of the bereaved.

Before they leave for the night, La shows us how to keep the fire banked in the woodstove so that the warmth will last through the night. Theo wakes up every couple of hours, and his wails subside only when I bring him to my breast. Outside the window there is nothing but the blackest night. David gets out of bed to poke at the fire in the stove and for a while, we have a roaring blaze, but then it starts to smoke and die out.

"This is fucked up," I say. "What are we doing with Theo here? It's insane."

"It's the mountains," David says with a smile. "Of course it's insane."

I laugh. What used to be scary and crazy for David has through familiarity and marriage become another home. He gets the mountains now. He understands the way time in New Mexico moves like honey on a cold morning. He thanks my mom for surrounding him with white light. He is as delighted as I am when our freezer is stocked with bags of Hatch green chile. He enjoys this life, but doesn't feel compelled to make it his own. I envy him this ability. I admire the easy way that he keeps a foot in both worlds and never feels like he is short changing one for the other.

"The cats are going to suffocate the baby," I say.

David heads outside to get more wood for the fire. I pull Theo's blanket around him and pace in the living room. I can't quiet my thoughts. That little bird is caught in my chest. Its wings are fluttering against my heart. I can't breathe. I can't feel.

Once, Dad and I spent a hot, rainy night in Dallas, Texas, camped out in the office of a factory where they manufactured amusement park rides. The office manager left the air conditioning on for us and apologized for having to lock us in. Dad said he didn't mind being locked in as long as it was cool. We unrolled our sleeping bags and tried to go to sleep, but someone had left a radio on. All night long, the radio broadcast reports on the flooding and on an area serial killer who was terrorizing the city. I tried to be brave, but eventually asked Dad if he thought we were going to be okay.

"Serial killers don't go out in the rain," Dad said. "Anyway, we're locked in so he's locked out. I'll stay awake and keep guard; you get some sleep."

Dad was always on guard. He kept me safe from werewolves, vampires, gargoyles, and witches. Once when I'd had a particularly bad dream, he brought in a crucifix, some garlic, a Crow Mother kachina, and the Star of David. He nailed each of these items in one corner of my room.

"There, we've got you covered. This place is powerfully protected. No matter who's coming, they're gonna run when they get here."

Dad is not here to protect me now. He is really gone.

I'm crying when David returns with an armload of wood. He drops the whole pile onto the floor and curves his arm around my shoulders.

"Shh," David says. "Shhh."

He leads me back to the bed and tucks the quilt up around Theo and me.

"I'm going to get the fire going," he says.

I nod. From the next room, I can hear the clang of fireplace tools. I can hear David exhale again and again, hoping to ignite a spark. Theo has gone back to sleep. He's wrapped like a burrito, his nose just visible above the edge of his blanket. I take deep breaths and scissor my legs against the sheets, warming the bed for my husband.

Good to Know You * *November 2002*

IN THE MINIATURE western village that is Tinkertown, past the hotel and the soda parlor, the blacksmith and the toyshop, the last thing you come to is Boot Hill cemetery. Dad set up a funeral in progress, complete with a few mourners in black and a crusty looking gravedigger. The lid of the casket pops open at intervals to reveal a tiny wood-carved figure of Dad. He's wearing blue jeans, his beard is red and trimmed and he's holding a paintbrush over his chest as if it were a rose.

"Who the hell else could I put in there?" he asked years ago, when he created the cemetery. "It just wouldn't be fair."

A tiny Corona beer bottle is glued to the lid of the casket next to a sign that invites you to "Have one on Ross." Just below the casket another sign reads, "So long, it's been good to know you."

It is the morning of the memorial and La has just returned from picking up Dad's ashes. She tells us that before Dad was cremated, the attendant asked if there were "any distinguishing marks" that could be used to identify the body.

"I looked at the woman and said, well, there are the big eyeballs tattooed on the tops of his feet . . ."

We laugh and begin to catalogue my father's distinguishing marks.

"There's a lizard running down each leg," my brother says.

"A circus poster on his shoulder," I say.

I think of his crooked thumbs, of the deep laugh lines around his eyes, and the way his hair curved up just above his collar. I think of his long, pale legs and the way his feet turned out when he walked. I think, too, of the distinguishing marks left on his brain by his disease, about the dark caves in tissue that was once bright with imagination and life. I grab La's rough hand in my own. She meets my eyes and squeezes hard.

Dad was put into a big cardboard box and sent into a furnace. With him were letters from La and my brother and because I was not there to write anything new, a Father's Day card I sent this past June. A day later, when he is returned to us, Dad fits in a brown cardboard cylinder a bit bigger than a gallon of ice cream. I am surprised by the weight of the container. Somehow I'd expected ashes to be light. The heft of my father in this new state is satisfying. It is oddly comforting to hold the box in my lap, curving my hands around the smooth side. On the lid, against a background of silver metal, is a label that confirms the identity of the "remains." My father's name has been typed out on a manual typewriter and the letters do not all sit in an even line. They've left out his middle initial. The canister is held together in the middle by a thick piece of clear packing tape. I run my fingernail gently over the tape along the seam where the two pieces of cardboard come together.

"Can we open him?" I ask La.

"I want to," she says. She sits on the couch next to me.

I press my fingernail harder against the tape and feel it give. I slide the lid off and look inside. The ashes are in a plastic bag held shut by a twist tie. As I undo the twist tie and open the bag, bits of dust drift out and sparkle in the sunlight. I am breathing bits of Dad. The ashes are the color and consistency of Redi-Mix mortar.

"He looks just like cement," I say.

As I say this, I can almost hear the scrape of a trowel hitting the inside of the old wheelbarrow. I can see Dad holding a bit of mortar in his hand, tucking it between two bottles. I can see him fitting a rock into the wall, gently scraping away the excess mortar.

"Let's mix up another tub of mud," he'd say, stepping back to admire his work. "Check that. It looks like a million bucks."

"Some people have asked if they could have a little bit of your dad," La says. "What would you think of that?"

"I think he'd like that," I say. "I think he'd like to go home with everyone here."

Months ago, at the urging of our friend Chris, La, Jason, Megan, David, and I got together to talk about Dad's funeral. Chris passed out notebooks with sparkly covers and opened a bottle of champagne.

"Let's just brainstorm," she said. "How do you do right by that old kook?"

Jason suggested we call it "The Great Pop Off" and we all laughed. We talked about music (Bob Dylan) and speeches (no weepy sentimentality), food (green chile cheeseburgers) and a guest list (family and close friends). We made some notes and promised to get things organized so that when the time came, we would be ready, but we didn't meet again.

Today, calls have been made to what La refers to as the usual suspects, including my uncle Louie, La's best friends Chris and Joni, my godmother Julie, my mom, Megan's parents. David's parents are flying in to say good-bye to my dad and hello to their new grandson. We have a huge pile of burgers ready to go on the grill and beer in the fridge. We are as ready as we'll ever be.

In a letter to me dated "Ape-ril—7th–8E7," Dad wrote, "Thank you for having the foresight on the great wheel of reincarnation to be my kid." He'd drawn lightning bolts and storm clouds in the margins of the three-hole paper, and numerous figures with stars on their cheeks asked, "But is this really?" The second page of the letter was nothing but shapes. At the bottom, he'd written, "Free at last from formal form!"

On the morning of the memorial, we put some of the ashes into an old Fixall enamel paint can that La unearths in the shop. The label describes the color within as "Mohawk Red." Megan has brought some small brown cardboard boxes for visitors to fill and she arranges them neatly on the wooden dresser that will function as a shrine. The boxes are the perfect size to fit in a pocket and are comforting to hold. I have already filled mine and tucked it into a zippered compartment in my suitcase.

"It's weird," La begins, "but I kind of wonder what he'll taste like."

"So taste him," my brother says.

La wets the tip of her finger and places it in the ashes while we all watch.

"Kind of like dirt," she says.

Jason and I lick our fingers almost simultaneously and take a taste.

"Pennies," I say.

"Beer?" Jason offers.

"All right, this is so strange," David says. "But I've got to do it now."

My husband wets his finger and tastes the ashes of my father. "Pretty salty," he says, "but then, that's no surprise."

"Dad is looking down on this and laughing his ass off," Jason says.

✳ ✳ ✳

Just before everyone begins to arrive, I change Theo's diaper. I massage his tiny legs and marvel again at how each of his toes is no bigger than a black bean. He likes being naked, and I let him bask in the sun that streams across the bed.

When I was living at Tinkertown, I spent a lot of time sitting on this bed in the sun, watching Dad flip through his scrapbooks. He'd kept these big, black bound books for years, adding news articles, brochures, and photographs, documenting everything he found interesting. As his Alzheimer's progressed, Dad's role as curator of these scrapbooks became more and more random. Open one and you might find a Roy Rogers obituary next to a flattened M&Ms bag. Ticket stubs from museums Dad visited mingled with photos and drawings and nudes torn from the pages of *Playboy*. He spent hours cutting things out and pasting them back in, eventually cannibalizing the scrapbooks themselves, layering images and articles one on top of another until the books were bloated at the bindings, so filled with information and history they could not close. The books were no longer a reference tool, but instead mirrored Dad's brain, which had become a jumble of the meaningful and the trivial with no clear line to divide the two.

I am pulling up Theo's soft, blue pants when the stump of his umbilical cord falls off. I hold it in my palm and am suddenly struck by the idea that we start to separate from our parents at the outset. The realization that this bit of dried skin and blood is the last thing that physically connects me to Theo breaks my heart, but it is his job to grow away from me. All I can do is make sure he's well equipped for the journey. I place the cord along with the plastic clamp that stopped the flow of blood into a second brown cardboard box and use a rubber band to secure it to the box holding my portion of Dad's ashes.

The party (for that's what it has turned out to be) is in full swing. Though we didn't put out any formal invitations, the parking lot is full, and cars line the road on both sides of our driveway. La, wearing a black sweater over a red turtleneck, greets the newly arrived and carries the latest tinfoil-wrapped offering to the kitchen counter. We are knee-deep in casseroles and cinnamon buns, but also, because this is Dad's party, the museum collection expands. Our friend Chris brings an empty beer bottle fitted with galvanized metal wings, Jon Schneck brings a drawing of Dad on horseback floating up over the carnival midway into the arms of a topless woman, and my uncle Louie offers a carefully painted sign inscribed with the dates marking Dad's life and the words, "I love you, honey, but the season's over." Flowers and hand-painted cards are added to a makeshift shrine where candles burn next to a bouquet of paintbrushes. Behind the candles is a black-and-white photo of Dad that was taken at my wedding. He is sitting at an iron table. The buttons on his woven Chimayo vest are undone and he is looking off to the side, his eyes crinkled with laughter.

On Sunday afternoons, when I was a kid, we used to go to the Golden Inn, a bar where a group of local musicians called The Watermelon Mountain Jug Band played regularly. While they rattled through "Rocky Top" or "You Are My Sunshine," the grown-ups all drank beer and Jason and I ran around with our friends, getting hopped up on sarsaparilla and practicing twirls on the dance floor. Because my parents knew everyone, there was always a hand on my shoulder or a wink from across the room. Every adult seemed to be an extension of my parents, just one more comforting strand in an invisible safety net. I had the freedom to pass through this space on my own, but somewhere, someone was always looking after me.

Today, as I wander through the crowd holding Theo, I have that same feeling. Many of these people held me when I was a child, and now everyone wants to hold my boy. I pass him gently into one set of open arms after another. My godmother, Julie, snuggles him against her bright turquoise flannel shirt.

"Hello there, young man," she says. She offers me a toothy grin despite her damp eyes. "Can you believe you were ever this small?"

My uncle Louie settles Theo into the crook of his arm. Though his two boys are well into their twenties, his body begins to rock automatically as if the small weight of my son has shifted his internal rhythm back to the early days of his own fatherhood.

"Sure is a good party," he says softly. "Ross would have enjoyed it."

It's true. It's a museum of people. There's no other way that gray-skinned Leon, the circus enthusiast who once brought a reel-to-reel tape recorder to preserve a revival screening of *The Greatest Show on Earth*, would be sharing space with an onyx-haired biker chick named Angel who used to tend bar down the road, but here we all are, eating green chile cheeseburgers and raising beers to the memory of my dad.

Night is coming on and the cottage is filling with people seeking warmth. I can smell smoke from the fire pit on their clothes. Jason wanders through the crowd holding a drowsy Hedy Rose. In her sparkly flowered dress and striped tights, she stands out like fireworks against his black shirt. Just outside the window, the big dark shape of the Sandias stands guard over our little doings. My boy is stirring in my arms, turning his face toward me looking for food, and I feel a tingling response as my milk comes in. I look down at his head. It's only a bit larger than my fist and yet inside, his brain is already set to record.

Several months ago, I dreamt that Dad had died. I have had this dream many times, and it usually ends quickly because I wake myself up by crying. But on this night, I let the dream continue. I had a feeling that something else was coming and, sure enough, after I cried a bit, a train pulled up and I climbed on board. Inside there was beautiful wood paneling, brass fittings, and rows and rows of crystal clear windows. I took a seat and stared out at the passing forest, losing myself in the green, until someone sat next to me. It was Dad. He gave me a minute to register his presence, the gold filling in his front tooth glimmering behind the beginning of a smile. I leaned against his shoulder.

"But they told me you were dead," I said.

"Aw, come on, Tanya, death's just bullshit, you know that."

With his warm presence behind me, I turned back to the window, back to the blur of trees and the bright blue sky.

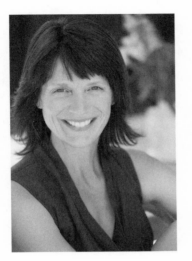

Tanya Ward Goodman lives in Los Angeles with her husband and two children.